EAT TO LIVE

QUICK & EASY COOKBOOK

Also by Joel Fuhrman

The End of Heart Disease

The End of Dieting

Eat to Live Cookbook

The End of Diabetes

Super Immunity

Eat for Health

Disease-Proof Your Child

Fasting and Eating for Health

Eat to Live

EAT TO LIVE

QUICK & EASY COOKBOOK

131 Delicious, Nutrient-Rich Recipes for Fast and Sustained
Weight Loss, Reversing Disease, and Lifelong Health

JOEL FUHRMAN, M.D.

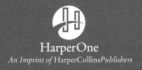

HarperOne
An Imprint of HarperCollinsPublishers

The results of any diet or medical intervention can vary from person to person. Some people have a medical history and/or condition that may warrant individualized recommendations and, in some cases, drugs and even surgery. Do not start, stop, or change your diet if you are ill or on medication except under the supervision of a competent physician. Neither this nor any other book is intended to take the place of personalized medical care or treatment.

HarperCollins books may be purchased for educational, business, or sales promotional use. For information, please email the Special Markets Department at SPsales@harpercollins.com.

FIRST EDITION

Designed by Kris Tobiassen of Matchbook Digital

Library of Congress Cataloging-in-Publication Data is available upon request.

ISBN 978–0–06–268495–0
ISBN 978–0–06–269642–7 (Costco edition)

17 18 19 20 21   LSC   10 9 8 7 6 5 4 3 2 1

Contents

EAT TO LIVE

QUICK & EASY COOKBOOK

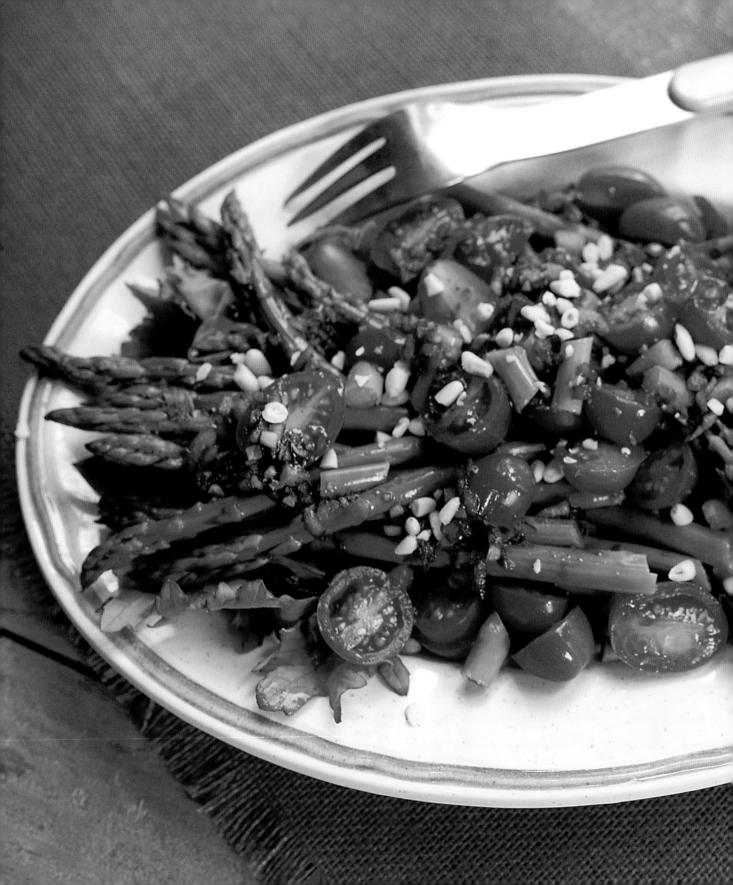

Introduction

Eating well does not have to be a time-consuming, labor-intensive process. I have compiled this collection of quick and easy recipes so that everyone, even those with very busy schedules or little inclination to cook, can follow a nutrient-rich diet for optimal health and disease prevention.

Diet plans come and go. Every year, new schemes appear that promise weight loss, renewed health, a glowing complexion, or enhanced longevity. But the truth is, there is only one answer—and it is very simple.

You must eat foods that supply your body with the nutrients it needs. There is no way around it. If you exist on a diet of refined, processed, nutrient-depleted fast foods, eventually you will pay the consequences. Obesity, diabetes, heart disease, many cancers, and other diseases can all be traced to poor nutrition, that is, a deficiency of vital nutrients and/or the overconsumption of foods that are harmful.

Eating healthfully is the single most effective preventive and therapeutic intervention available. It is the best way to maintain a favorable long-term weight, and it is the best "prescription" any doctor can give you.

For more than twenty-five years, I have helped tens of thousands of people gain control over their health and weight with a Nutritarian diet. A Nutritarian diet is not designed to be popular or trendy, but instead to be the healthiest and most lifespan-enhancing diet style possible. The word *Nutritarian* means a diet that is rich in plant-derived micronutrients—particularly antioxidants and phytochemicals—and that utilizes foods that offer proven anticancer protection. Lasting health and permanent weight loss are not unattainable goals. They are within reach when you learn to choose the right foods. A high-nutrient diet that is rich in vegetables slows the aging process,

> A nutrient-dense, plant-rich diet is effective for long-term weight control, because you feel full and satisfied even when you are consuming fewer calories.

enables repair of cell damage, reduces inflammation, and helps rid the body of toxins. Meeting your body's nutrient needs also helps to suppress the hunger and cravings that fuel the overeating of low-nutrient, high-calorie, refined, processed foods.

Natural plant foods contain thousands of nutrients, many that have been discovered and others that are presently unidentified, so it is important to consume an adequate amount, and a wide variety, of these foods. These plant-derived nutrients are valuable in protecting against later-life cancer, as well as protecting the aging brain against dementia.

Whole plant foods, with their nature-given, fragile phytonutrients, should comprise the majority of your diet. The great-tasting recipes in this book feature the healthiest foods on the planet and make it easy for you to build your menus around them. I've selected these recipes because they require a minimal amount of time and preparation. Some are easy, and some are very easy. I'm sure you will enjoy many of them and will want to make them again and again.

To your good health!

JOEL FUHRMAN, M.D.

The Nutritarian Lifestyle

Most people are misinformed about food and healthful eating. They drift from one fad diet to another, without ever understanding the bigger picture. I believe in teaching my patients and readers to be experts in nutrition so that they have the keys to health and successful weight control in their hands.

If you have read any of my books, such as *Eat to Live, The End of Dieting,* or *The End of Heart Disease,* you know that the secret to eating well is to focus on micronutrients, not calories. Eating healthfully and consuming the right assortment and amount of nutrients results in consistent, long-term health benefits. Getting healthy and maintaining a stable, appropriate weight can be achieved only by paying attention to the nutritional quality of your food for the rest of your life.

What you eat determines your weight more than *how much* you eat.

People who follow a Nutritarian diet recognize that plant foods have disease-preventive, therapeutic, and life-extending properties. If you are overweight, this diet will enable you to lose weight and keep it off permanently, without experiencing hunger or feeling deprived, because it is based on eating large quantities of satisfying, nutritious foods.

Some of you may find that it takes some time for your taste buds to become more sensitive and your food preferences to change. You may be used to high-salt, high-sugar, and high-fat foods. However, with time, most people find that they actually prefer the taste of Nutritarian foods.

Knowledge trumps willpower every time.

I am hopeful that you will enjoy this way of eating. I know that you'll like the way you feel, and—best of all—that you'll love being free from chronic disease and the constant yo-yo dieting that make life miserable for so many Americans. The results of the Nutritarian eating style are sustainable, because once people become nutritional experts and experience success, they want to eat this way forever. The secret to success is knowledge: The more you learn, the easier it becomes to eat this way for the rest of your life.

Basic Guidelines of a Nutritarian Diet Style

Do the following every day:

1. Eat a large salad as the main dish for at least one meal.

2. Eat one large serving of cooked green vegetables.

3. Eat at least half a cup of beans.

4. Eat at least three servings of fresh or frozen fruit.

5. Eat at least 1 ounce of nuts and seeds if you're female and at least 1 ½ ounces if you're male. Half of this quantity should be walnuts, hemp seeds, chia seeds, flaxseeds, or sesame seeds.

6. Eat some cooked mushrooms and a combination of raw and cooked onions and tomatoes.

Eat few, if any, animal products (meat, fish, dairy, and eggs) and limit them to two or three small servings per week. Avoid red meat and all barbecued, processed, and cured meats. Animal products are restricted on a Nutritarian diet for many reasons, but mostly because higher amounts of animal protein in the diet are linked to higher levels of insulin-like growth factor-1 (IGF-1) and higher rates of cancer.

A Nutritarian diet is relatively high in plant protein because it is rich in green vegetables, beans, nuts, and seeds. Plant protein does not raise IGF-1 to unfavorable levels. Nutritarians generally prefer to use very small amounts of animal products, if any at all. When they do eat animal products, the animal products are used as condiments, to add flavor to stews or soups or wokked vegetable dishes, but they do not make the animal product a major caloric contributor to the meal.

In this book, I show you creative ways to use a very small amount—typically, just 1 ounce of animal product per serving—to add a meaty flavor and texture to veggie-based dishes. And for people who prefer not to eat animal products, some of those recipes offer vegan substitutions.

Whether you eat a little bit of animal products or none at all, the most important focus of a Nutritarian diet is to avoid foods that are empty of nutrients or are toxic to the body, such as sugar, sweeteners (including honey, agave nectar, and maple syrup), white flour, white rice, and other processed, refined foods.

Build Your Diet on a Foundation of Vegetables

Eat a salad every day, and make it extra large. Include lettuce, tomatoes, chopped onion, and at least one shredded cruciferous vegetable. Use a variety of greens, including

- Romaine lettuce
- Butter, Boston, or Bibb lettuce
- Red or green leaf lettuce
- Arugula
- Baby spinach
- Watercress
- Mâche

For added veggies, choose from red or green bell peppers, cucumbers, carrots, shredded red or green cabbage, chopped white or red onions, lightly sautéed mushrooms, zucchini, raw and lightly steamed beets and carrots, snow peas, broccoli, cauliflower, and radishes. Use the healthy nut- and seed-based dressings featured in this book to top off your salad. The fat from the nuts and seeds will help you absorb the nutrients in the vegetables.

It is best to include both raw and cooked vegetables. The levels of some nutrients are higher in raw vegetables, but others are made more available by cooking. In addition to your salad, eat a hearty portion of cooked vegetables each day. Great choices include cooked leafy greens, such as kale, collards, mustard greens, bok choy, and spinach; and broccoli, Brussels sprouts, asparagus, cabbage, and zucchini.
I like to simmer vegetables in a soup because all the nutrients are retained in the cooking liquid. I also gently steam or water-sauté veggies in many of my recipes.

While all vegetables contain protective micronutrients and phytochemicals, cruciferous vegetables have especially powerful anticancer effects. Try to include vegetables from this family in your diet every day. Kale, collards, mustard greens, arugula, cabbage, bok choy, broccoli, Brussels sprouts, and cauliflower are all cruciferous vegetables. They contain compounds called *glucosinolates* and, in a different area of the cell, an enzyme called *myrosinase*. When cruciferous vegetables are blended, chopped, or

> Green vegetables are the secret weapon to fight almost all diseases. Add greens to everything.

chewed, the plant cell walls are broken, allowing myrosinase to come into contact with glucosinolates. This initiates a chemical reaction that produces *isothiocyanates,* which have been shown to detoxify and remove carcinogens.

Magic Beans

Beans and other legumes, such as lentils and split peas, are the ideal starchy foods because they have uniquely high levels of fiber and *resistant starch,* that is, carbohydrates that are not broken down by the digestive system. Because these carbohydrates are indigestible, the calories from them do not count. You can eat high-nutrient, low-calorie beans in large quantities without any danger of gaining weight. Their fiber and resistant starch contents make them very satiating, allowing you to feel full longer and fight off food cravings.

Fiber and resistant starch limit the glycemic (blood sugar–raising) effects of beans, making them an ideal food for preventing or reversing diabetes. In addition, when these compounds reach your colon, they act as food for your healthy gut bacteria. This promotes the formation of compounds that protect against colon cancer.

> Beans are among the world's most perfect foods. They stabilize blood sugar, blunt the desire for sweets, and prevent between-meal cravings.

Try to eat at least half a cup of beans, lentils, or split peas every day. Add them to your salad; include them in soups, stews, or chili; make bean burgers or blend them into dips for raw vegetables. Enjoy a wide variety of beans, including chickpeas, black beans, red kidney beans, cannellini beans, soybeans, black-eyed peas, pinto beans, lentils, and split peas. In this book, I show you how to prepare them in many different ways, using a wide variety of seasonings and spices. If you use canned beans for convenience, be sure to choose those that are low in sodium or have no salt added.

Naturally Sweet and Juicy Fruit

Always keep a good supply of fresh fruit on hand. It is the ultimate convenience food, and it is an excellent nutrient-dense, low-calorie source of vitamins and phytochemicals.

Every kind of fruit offers its own special benefits. Berries, in particular, are true superfoods, with extremely high antioxidant values. Their deep red, blue, and purple pigments are produced by *anthocyanins,* which are flavonoid compounds that have been associated with numerous health benefits. Anthocyanins have been linked to lower blood pressure levels and a reduced risk of diabetes, as well as improved memory and motor coordination.

Frozen fruit is a good quick and easy option. Keep your freezer stocked with a variety of choices. The nutritional value of frozen fruit is comparable to that of fresh fruit. But avoid canned fruit because it often has added sweeteners and has lost a significant amount of its water-soluble nutrients.

As regards dried fruit, use it only in small amounts as a sweetener in recipes if you need to lose weight.

Shoot for three servings of fruit a day, including one serving of berries. Enjoy strawberries, blueberries, raspberries, or blackberries stirred into your morning oatmeal, added to a smoothie, or as a simple dessert.

> Fruit, consumed at its peak of ripeness, is more delicious than any processed, overrefined dessert or treat.

The Good Fats: Seeds and Nuts

Fat provides the essential fatty acids linoleic and linolenic acid, which are called "essential" because your body cannot make them and cannot remain healthy without them. These essential fatty acids are needed for brain development, the control of inflammation, and the clotting of blood. Fat helps to keep your skin healthy and is required for the absorption of the fat-soluble vitamins A, D, E, and K.

It is well known that the saturated fats in animal products such as butter, cheese, whole milk, ice cream, and meats should be avoided. They raise low-density lipoprotein (LDL) cholesterol ("bad" cholesterol), which puts you at risk for heart attack, stroke, and other major health problems. But you should also skip refined vegetable oils, including olive oil. Like sugar, vegetable oils are processed foods that have had almost all of their nutrients and fiber removed. Ounce for ounce, oil is one of the most calorically dense foods you can eat, which adds up to a lot of empty calories.

Nuts and seeds are the healthful alternatives to olive oil. They are rich in fiber, protein, sterols, minerals, lignans, and other health-promoting nutrients, and they increase the absorption of nutrients from other foods as well. The fats in nuts and seeds are slowly absorbed, so they keep you feeling full for a longer time. Researchers have found that including nuts and seeds in your diet can help you lose weight and can also protect against heart disease and cancer.

Eat nuts and seeds raw or just lightly toasted, because the roasting process alters their beneficial fats. Commercially packaged nuts and seeds are frequently cooked in oil and are heavily salted.

> In a nutshell, seeds and nuts are the best source of healthy fats.

If you are trying to lose weight, limit nuts and seeds to 1 ounce (about ¼ cup) for women and 1 ½ ounces for men. If you are active and slim, there is no problem with eating more than this. At least half of your nut intake should be walnuts, hemp seeds, chia seeds, flaxseeds, or sesame seeds, because all of these (except sesame) are particularly high in essential omega-3 fats. In addition, all (except walnuts) are excellent sources of lignans, which reduce cholesterol and provide extra protection against cancer.

People with nut allergies can substitute pumpkin seeds, sunflower seeds, or sunflower seed butter in recipes calling for cashews, almonds, or other nuts. Unhulled sesame seeds or raw tahini are also tasty options, but because they are stronger in flavor, start off with a lower amount and adjust according to taste.

Toss out your empty-calorie, refined oils and use a high-powered blender to make creamy dressings from nuts and seeds. These dressings will taste great, you'll absorb more nutrients from the veggies, thanks to the healthy fats, and you'll feel full longer.

Don't Forget to Add Mushrooms, Onions, and Tomatoes

Mushrooms have tremendous powers to enhance your immune system function. All types of mushrooms have a wide variety of anticancer properties. They are *antiangiogenic,* which means they inhibit the growth of abnormal cells, tumors, and cancers. Eating even a small amount of mushrooms each day will help protect you against cancer. As a safety precaution, always cook your mushrooms, since some animal studies have reported toxic effects of raw mushrooms.

> **Allium vegetables include onions, garlic, leeks, chives, shallots, and scallions. They are rich in cancer-fighting organosulfur compounds. An increased consumption of these vegetables is associated with a decreased risk of many types of cancers.**

The *Allium* genus of vegetables—onions, garlic, leeks, chives, shallots, and scallions—does more than just add great flavor to meals. These vegetables are anti-diabetic and anticancer foods and have beneficial effects on the cardiovascular and immune systems. Use them generously in your cooking. To gain their full benefits, eat them raw and chew them well, or blend or chop them finely before cooking to initiate the chemical reaction that forms protective sulfur compounds.

Tomatoes are a rich source of *lycopene,* a carotenoid pigment linked to reduced risk of cancer, heart disease, and age-related eye disorders. Add tomatoes to your salad, and enjoy them in soups, stews, and sauces. Choose low-sodium or no-salt-added tomato products, and, to minimize exposure to the endocrine disruptor bisphenol-A (BPA), look for tomato products packaged in glass or cartons instead of in cans. Lycopene is more absorbable when tomatoes are cooked, so enjoy a variety of both raw and cooked tomatoes.

To help you remember the superfoods you should include in your diet every day, think G-BOMBS:

Greens Beans Onions Mushrooms Berries Seeds

What About Grains?

Grain products are not as nutrient dense as vegetables and fruit, so they should make up a smaller portion of your diet. Limit them to one to two servings daily. Stick with whole grain products, preferably intact whole grains. Refined grains such as white pasta, white rice, and bread products made from white flour lose a big part of their nutrient value during processing. You should avoid them completely.

Intact whole grains are the best choice because they consist of the whole grain that has not been ground up and so still contains the fiber-rich hull. Intact whole grains include steel cut oats, buckwheat, quinoa, millet, barley (not pearled), farro, and wheat berries.

The whiter the bread, the sooner you're dead.

When choosing a whole grain bread, pita, or wrap, make sure it is 100 percent whole grain. Read the ingredient list; a whole grain should be the first ingredient. If more than one grain is used, they should all be whole grains. Be aware that just because a bread item claims to be "multigrain" or "whole wheat," this does not mean it is made with 100 percent whole grains.

Bread products made with sprouted grains are a good option. Wheat kernels, as well as other grains such as millet, barley, and oats, are allowed to sprout and are then ground up and baked into the bread. Because these grains are coarsely ground, they have an improved nutrient and glycemic profile.

No Room for Processed Sweeteners, White Flour, or Oils

Why are more than two-thirds of Americans overweight or obese? Why has the prevalence of obesity among adults more than doubled in the past fifty years? The root of the problem is that the Standard American Diet (SAD) now contains lots and lots of calories, but few nutrients.

If you are 100 percent committed, you always find a way to make it work.

Sugary drinks, baked goods, fried foods, refined grain products, and salty snacks are all to blame. They are made with ingredients like white flour, white sugar, and oils that are so processed and refined that no real nutritional value is left in them. These excessively sweet, salty, and/or fatty foods are engineered to be so highly palatable that they can have addictive effects in the human brain, driving loss of self-control, overeating, and weight gain. The top two sources of calories in the SAD are grain-based desserts (cakes, cookies, donuts, pies) and bread.

> Side effects of the Nutritarian diet include improving your overall health, feeling more energetic, and losing weight effortlessly.

Avoid products made with empty-calorie ingredients. Sticking with natural whole foods that are unprocessed or minimally processed is a key step in reaching and maintaining your ideal body weight and reducing your risk of diabetes, heart disease, and cancer.

Cooking Techniques and Tips

Steaming Is Quick and Easy

Steaming vegetables couldn't be any easier. You need only a steamer pot with a lid, or a steamer basket to place in a pot with a lid. Add a small amount of water to the bottom of the pot (about an inch), keeping the water level below the bottom of the steamer basket.

Note: Don't steam vegetables until they are very soft. If you do, you will lose many of the water-soluble nutrients.

Cut vegetables into similar-sized pieces and place in a steamer basket. Get the water boiling first, then add the vegetables, cover, and start a timer. I find that the times listed here work best; however, the less you cook greens, the more nutrients are retained.

Artichokes (cut in half and prepped)	18 minutes
Asparagus	10 minutes
Bok choy	10 minutes
Broccoli (stems sliced)	13 minutes
Brussels sprouts	13 minutes
Cabbage (sliced)	13 minutes
Cauliflower	14 minutes
Kale, collards, Swiss chard	10 minutes
Snow peas	10 minutes
Spinach	3–5 minutes
String beans	13 minutes
Zucchini	10 minutes

Sauté with Water Instead of Oil

Instead of adding unnecessary refined, empty-calorie oil to a recipe, I use a technique called *water-sautéing*. You will find that many of the recipes in this book begin with water-sautéing onions, garlic, or other vegetables.

Add a small amount of water (1–2 tablespoons) to a skillet or pan. Heat until water starts to steam. Add your vegetables and cook, stirring frequently. Allow the pan to dry out just enough for the food to start to brown a little before you add additional water as needed. This helps to develop the flavor in your ingredients without the addition of oil. You can alternately cover and stir to reduce the cooking time.

Mushrooms naturally contain a lot of water, which is released as they cook. They can be sautéed in their own juices, so there's no need to start out with water. Simply heat a dry pan over medium heat and then add sliced or chopped mushrooms. To avoid burning, stir frequently until the natural juices that are released are evaporated.

Blend Up Some Amazing Dressings, Dips, and Desserts

Smoothies and blended salads make a quick, easy, and portable option for breakfast or lunch. Blend together raw leafy green vegetables, fruits, seeds, and nuts for a to-go meal that you can eat quickly. The blender crushes the cell walls of the plants more efficiently than chewing, making it easier for your body to absorb the beneficial phytochemicals that are locked inside the plants' cells.

Nut- and seed-based salad dressings and dips are an essential component of the Nutritarian diet. By blending nuts and seeds with other ingredients such as fruit, vinegar, and seasonings, you can make delicious dressings that enhance both the taste and the nutritional quality of your salads. And in addition to dressings and dips, some of my most

A durable, high-powered blender is an essential kitchen appliance for making my smoothies, salad dressings, vegetable dips, and creamy desserts. Because I use whole food ingredients such as vegetables, fruits, nuts, seeds, and dried fruit, it is important that the machine have enough power and speed to efficiently process these ingredients to the desired smooth consistency. Inexpensive models will not provide a nice, creamy texture, and their motors tend to burn out after a month or two of daily use. Add a bit more water or liquid to the recipe if your blender is having problems keeping up.

popular soups are made by blending raw nuts into the soup to provide a creamy texture and rich flavor.

Here's some good news: You don't need to banish dessert from your life! A good blender helps you create refreshing fruit sorbets and ice creams (which I frequently relabel "nice creams") by blending simple combinations of healthful ingredients such as fruit and nuts. I take pride in creating recipes for delicious and nutrient-rich cakes, pies, and cookies. Just you wait and taste!

Use Herbs, Spices, and Seasonings

Instead of adding salt, sugar, fat, and extra calories to your foods, season them with spices and fresh or dried herbs to enhance flavor. Dried basil, rosemary, thyme, and oregano are all spice rack staples that can quickly boost the flavor of a recipe. Chili powder will add a kick to any dish, so add it to stews and chilies. Including a pinch (or more, if you like) of crushed red pepper flakes, or ground red pepper such as cayenne, will add a touch of heat and another dimension to a recipe. To get the most flavor out of dried herbs, crush them or rub them between your fingers before adding them to a dish.

It doesn't take a whole lot more time and effort to use fresh parsley, basil, dill, and cilantro instead of their dried versions. Add fresh herbs at the end of cooking for maximum flavor.

Most supermarkets now sell fresh herbs conveniently packaged in small amounts.

Parsley
The mild flavor of parsley complements many dishes. Incorporate it into your recipe or sprinkle it on top.

Basil
Fresh basil is a staple of Italian cooking and is a great addition to tomatoes.

Dill
Dill complements cucumbers, green beans, and many vegetable dishes.

Cilantro
Cilantro adds distinctive flavor to Mexican dishes like salsa and chili, as well as Asian curries.

The general rule of thumb is that 1 teaspoon of dried herbs equals 1 tablespoon of fresh.

Sprinkle cinnamon on fruit or oatmeal, or add it to soups and stews. Shake a bit on your carrots or squash to enhance their natural sweetness. Look for Ceylon cinnamon, which is known as "true cinnamon." In the United States, it's more common to find cassia cinnamon, a closely related and less expensive variety that contains high levels of coumarin, a naturally occurring substance that has the potential to damage the liver in high doses.

Vinegar and citrus ingredients, such as lemon, lime, and orange, enhance the flavors of a variety of dishes. They activate the same taste receptors as salt. Add a splash of fresh-squeezed lemon or lime juice at the end of the cooking time to balance and brighten your soup. Flavored vinegars can infuse your salads and cooked dishes with bright, bold flavors without adding oil, salt, or sugar. Try sherry vinegar, champagne vinegar, and good-quality balsamic vinegar. Experiment with a variety of fruit-flavored vinegars such as fig, orange, pear, or pomegranate.

For a savory, cheesy flavor, try using unfortified nutritional yeast—a deactivated yeast that is not the same as brewer's yeast, which is a product of the beer-making industry. Just a tablespoon or two of unfortified nutritional yeast can enhance soups, sauces, and dressings. Choose a nutritional yeast that is not fortified with folic acid. Some troubling studies have connected folic acid supplementation with breast, prostate, and colorectal cancers.

Because some of these items may be difficult to find at your local supermarket, I make them available on my website, www.drfuhrman.com. In addition to Ceylon cinnamon, a variety of delicious flavored vinegars, unfortified nutritional yeast, and natural cocoa powder, you will also find my no-salt seasoning blends VegiZest and MatoZest.

The evidence is irrefutable:

1. Vegetables, beans, nuts, seeds, and fruit are health-promoting foods.

2. Excessive amounts of animal products increase chronic disease.

3. Refined carbohydrates promote chronic disease and lead to people becoming overweight and obese.

RECIPES

BREAKFAST

*A healthy breakfast doesn't have to
be time consuming and complicated.*

It can be as simple as combining fresh, in-season fruit or thawed frozen fruit with your favorite raw nuts and seeds. Whole, intact grains such as steel cut oats or buckwheat, combined with fruit, nuts, and seeds, also make an easy and satisfying go-to breakfast, and keep you filled up until lunchtime. If you are rushed for time in the morning, prepare your breakfast the night before and have it ready and waiting in the refrigerator. Whole grains, seeds, and dried fruits are best enjoyed after a good overnight soak to soften them, so making the night before is not just a time saver, but also the healthiest and most tasty way to prepare your morning whole grain cereals.

It's okay to break with tradition. Increase the nutrient density of your diet by including vegetables or beans in your morning menu. You can enjoy a leftover bowl of soup for breakfast or some romaine lettuce leaves spread with bean dip or raw cashew or almond butter.

Many active people find it important to eat a substantial breakfast, but if you are not hungry or have lower caloric needs, it's fine to skip breakfast and enjoy an early lunch.

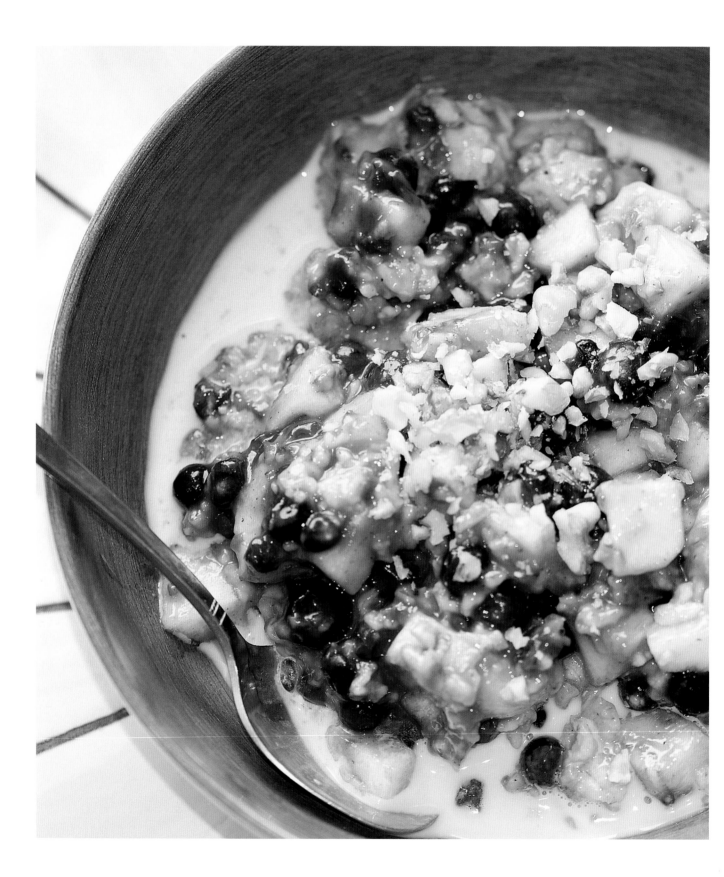

Blue Apple Nut Oatmeal

In a saucepan, combine the water, cinnamon, oats, and currants. Simmer until the oatmeal is creamy.

Add the blueberries and banana.

Cook for 5 minutes, or until hot, stirring constantly. Mix in the apple and nuts.

SERVES 2

1 ½ cups water

¼ teaspoon cinnamon

⅓ cup old-fashioned or steel cut oats*

2 tablespoons raisins or currants

1 cup fresh or frozen blueberries

1 banana, sliced

1 apple, peeled, cored, and chopped or grated

2 tablespoons chopped walnuts

....

If you use steel cut oats, increase cooking time to 20 minutes or until oats are tender.

TIP: Steel cut oats (also called Scotch or Irish oats) are a great choice because they are less processed than other oats. Instead of being steamed and rolled, oat groats are simply cut into pieces. They take longer to cook and have a chewy consistency. If you are in a rush, rolled oats (old-fashioned oats) require less cooking time. Do not use quick oats or instant oats because they are too highly refined and have lost a good portion of their nutrients.

PER SERVING: CALORIES 236; PROTEIN 4g; CARBOHYDRATES 51g; TOTAL FAT 4.2g; SATURATED FAT 0.5g; SODIUM 10mg; FIBER 6.7g; BETA-CAROTENE 57mcg; VITAMIN C 16mg; CALCIUM 32mg; IRON 4.2mg; FOLATE 21mcg; MAGNESIUM 36mg; ZINC 0.5mg; SELENIUM 0.9mcg

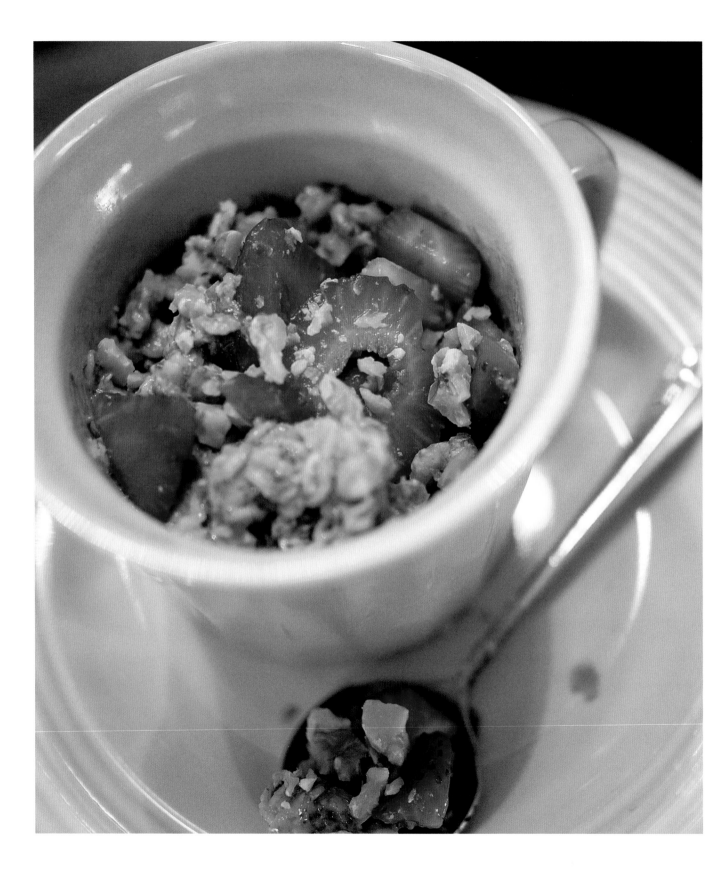

No-Cook Strawberry Oatmeal To-Go

You do have time for breakfast. Prepare this oatmeal the night before, and in the morning, you'll be ready to roll.

Place the oats and chia seeds in a portable cup. Add nondairy milk, and refrigerate overnight.

In the morning, stir in sliced strawberries and walnuts.

⅓ cup old-fashioned or steel cut oats

1 tablespoon chia seeds

⅔ cup unsweetened soy, hemp, or almond milk

1 cup fresh or thawed frozen strawberries, sliced*

6 walnut halves, crushed

* *You can also use blueberries, cherries, or sliced peaches.*

TIP: Berries are especially rich in beneficial phytochemical compounds. They have the highest nutrient-to-calorie ratio of all fruits.

PER SERVING: CALORIES 334; PROTEIN 13g; CARBOHYDRATES 39g; TOTAL FAT 16g; SATURATED FAT 1.8g; SODIUM 64mg; FIBER 11g; BETA-CAROTENE 13mcg; VITAMIN C 98mg; CALCIUM 306mg; IRON 9.2mg; FOLATE 52mcg; MAGNESIUM 100mg; ZINC 1.7mg; SELENIUM 6.8mcg

Cinnamon-Spiced Baked Oatmeal

SERVES 3

1 cup old-fashioned oats

⅓ cup raisins or chopped, unsulfured dried apricots

2 dates, chopped

2 tablespoons ground flaxseeds

1 cup unsweetened soy, hemp, or almond milk

⅔ cup water

1 teaspoon alcohol-free vanilla extract

1 teaspoon cinnamon or pumpkin pie spice

½ cup fresh or thawed frozen blueberries or other fruit

Preheat oven to 350°F.

Mix the oats, dried fruit, dates, flaxseeds, nondairy milk, water, vanilla, and spices in a mixing bowl, then place in a small baking dish.

For a 3-by-6-inch baking dish, bake 20–25 minutes or until most of the liquid is absorbed and the oats are golden brown. If using a larger baking dish, reduce the baking time.

After baking, top with blueberries. Serve hot or cold.

PER SERVING: CALORIES 311; PROTEIN 11g; CARBOHYDRATES 46g; TOTAL FAT 10.9g; SATURATED FAT 1.7g; SODIUM 49mg; FIBER 6.6g; BETA-CAROTENE 11mcg; VITAMIN C 3mg; CALCIUM 54mg; IRON 8.9mg; FOLATE 28mcg; MAGNESIUM 112mg; ZINC 1.2mg; SELENIUM 6.4mcg

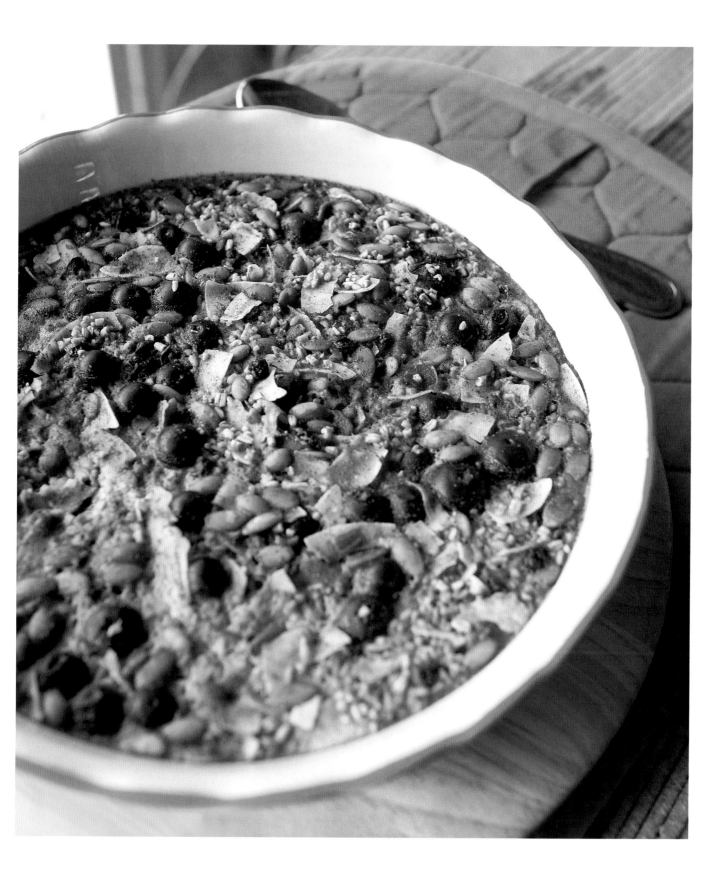

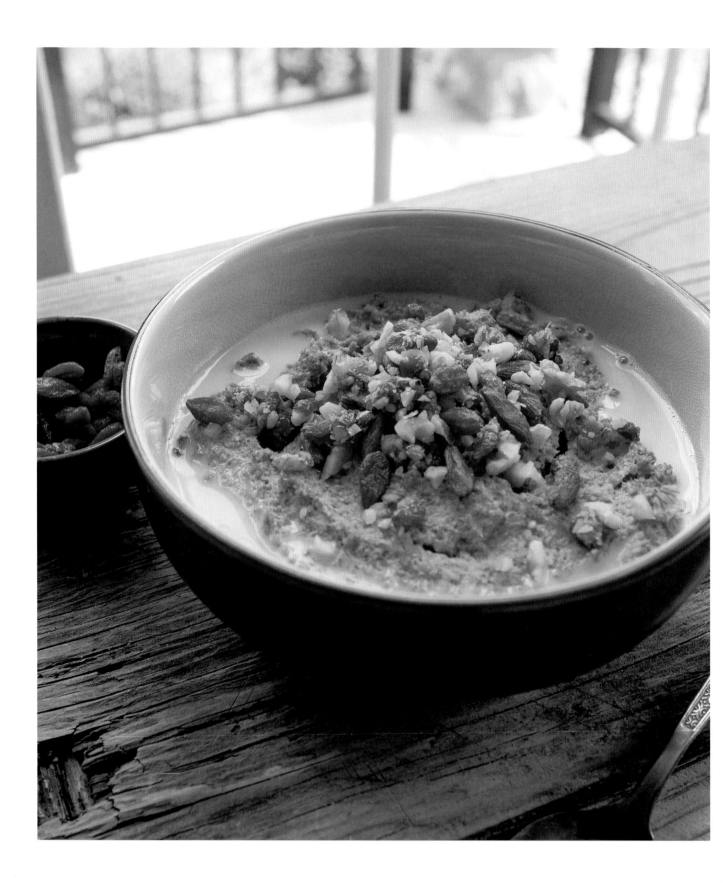

Creamy Buckwheat Porridge

Buckwheat groats are seeds from the buckwheat plant. They are unrelated to wheat and do not contain gluten. Choose raw buckwheat groats, not kasha, which is toasted.

Soak buckwheat groats overnight in 2 cups of water.

The next morning, drain and rinse.

Place buckwheat, dates, nondairy milk, vanilla, cinnamon, and chia seeds in a food processor and blend until smooth. Add additional nondairy milk if needed to achieve a creamy consistency.

Top with nuts and fresh fruit. Leftover cereal may be refrigerated; it will keep for several days.

SERVES 3

1 cup raw buckwheat groats

4 regular dates or 2 medjool dates, pitted

3 tablespoons unsweetened soy, hemp, or almond milk, or more as needed

1 teaspoon alcohol-free vanilla or almond extract

½ teaspoon cinnamon

1 teaspoon chia seeds

2 tablespoons chopped walnuts or other raw nuts

½ cup fresh or thawed frozen berries or other fruit

TIP: Buckwheat is rich in protein and fiber and has been shown to lower cholesterol. Kasha is toasted buckwheat and has a stronger flavor and darker color.

PER SERVING: CALORIES 305; PROTEIN 10g; CARBOHYDRATES 61g; TOTAL FAT 5g; SATURATED FAT 0.7g; SODIUM 10mg; FIBER 8.9g; BETA-CAROTENE 124mcg; VITAMIN C 4mg; CALCIUM 56mg; IRON 2mg; FOLATE 26mcg; MAGNESIUM 162mg; ZINC 1.7mg; SELENIUM 6.2mcg

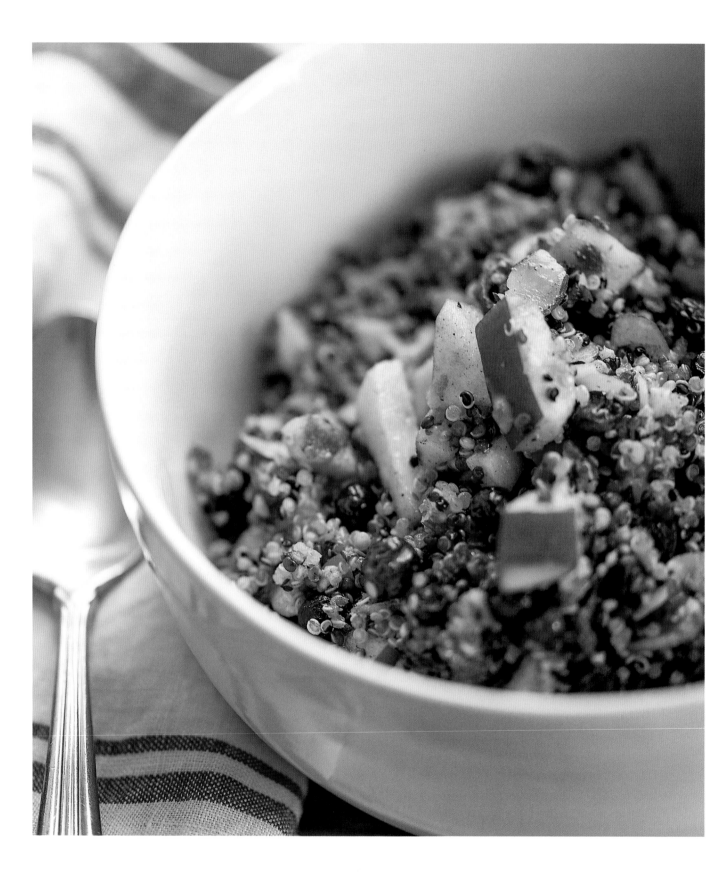

Quick Breakfast Quinoa

Place quinoa and water in a saucepan, bring to a boil, cover, reduce heat, and simmer for 15 minutes or until quinoa is done and all the water is absorbed. Fluff with a fork.

Add remaining ingredients and stir for 2–3 minutes.

SERVES 4

1 cup dry quinoa

2 cups water

1 medium apple, cored and diced

½ cup raw almonds, chopped

1 cup fresh or thawed frozen blueberries

½ cup raisins or chopped, pitted dates

1 teaspoon cinnamon

½ cup unsweetened soy, hemp, or almond milk

PER SERVING: CALORIES 332; PROTEIN 10g; CARBOHYDRATES 57g; TOTAL FAT 9.1g; SATURATED FAT 0.8g; SODIUM 33mg; FIBER 7.8g; BETA-CAROTENE 30mcg; VITAMIN C 4mg; CALCIUM 140mg; IRON 3mg; FOLATE 90mcg; MAGNESIUM 129mg; ZINC 1.8mg; SELENIUM 4.1mcg

Berry "Yogurt"

2 cups fresh or frozen
blueberries, blackberries,
or strawberries

¾ cup unsweetened soy, almond,
or hemp milk

2 tablespoons chia seeds

4 regular dates or 2 medjool
dates, pitted

Add all ingredients to a high-powered blender and blend until smooth. Chill before serving.

May be served with fresh or thawed frozen berries.

PER SERVING: CALORIES 238; PROTEIN 6g; CARBOHYDRATES 47g;
TOTAL FAT 5.1g; SATURATED FAT 0.5g; SODIUM 51mg; FIBER 7.5g;
BETA-CAROTENE 71mcg; VITAMIN C 14mg; CALCIUM 65mg; IRON 1.6mg;
FOLATE 35mcg; MAGNESIUM 72mg; ZINC 0.8mg; SELENIUM 6.3mcg

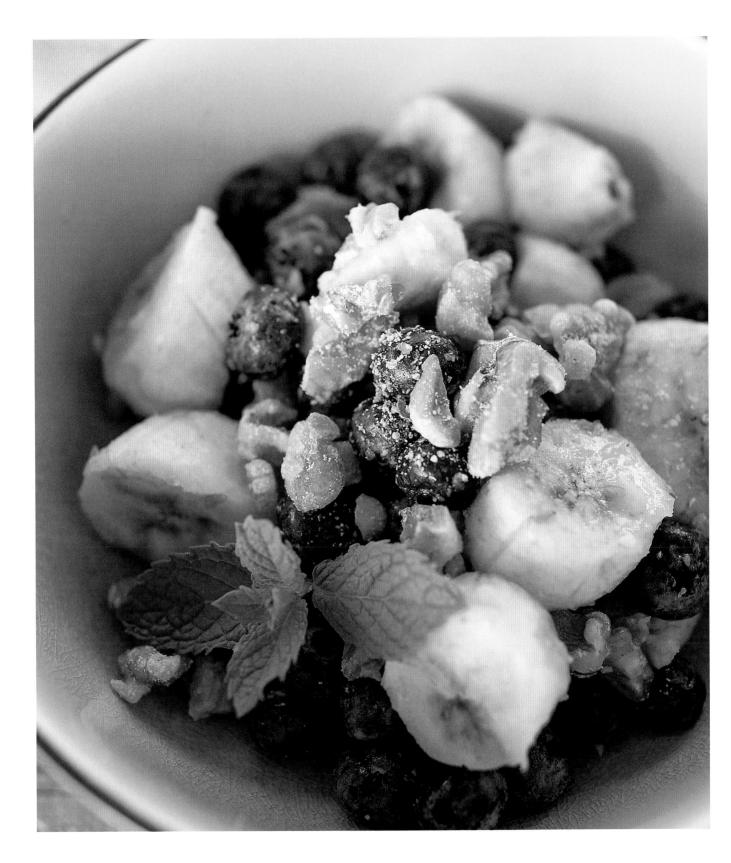

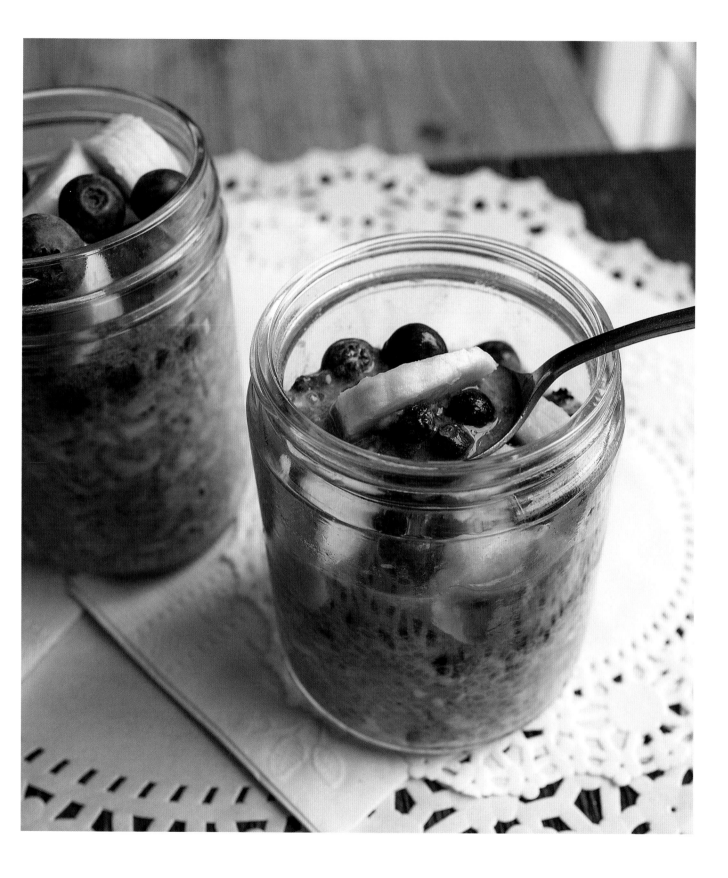

Chia Seed Breakfast Pudding

SERVES 1

½ cup unsweetened vanilla soy, almond, or hemp milk

2 tablespoons whole chia seeds

2 tablespoons old-fashioned oats

½ banana, sliced

½ cup fresh blueberries or frozen, thawed

Chia seeds are high in omega-3 fatty acids and fiber. They also have unique gelling properties, which make them perfect for making pudding.

In a bowl, mix together nondairy milk, chia seeds, and oats. Let mixture sit for 10 minutes. (For an on-the-run breakfast, make the night before and store in the refrigerator.)

Stir in banana and blueberries. Add additional nondairy milk if desired to adjust consistency.

PER SERVING: CALORIES 293; PROTEIN 10g; CARBOHYDRATES 46g; TOTAL FAT 9.7g; SATURATED FAT 1.1g; SODIUM 67mg; FIBER 12.1g; BETA-CAROTENE 39mcg; VITAMIN C 7mg; CALCIUM 166mg; IRON 5.1mg; FOLATE 39mcg; MAGNESIUM 117mg; ZINC 1.2mg; SELENIUM 17.6mcg

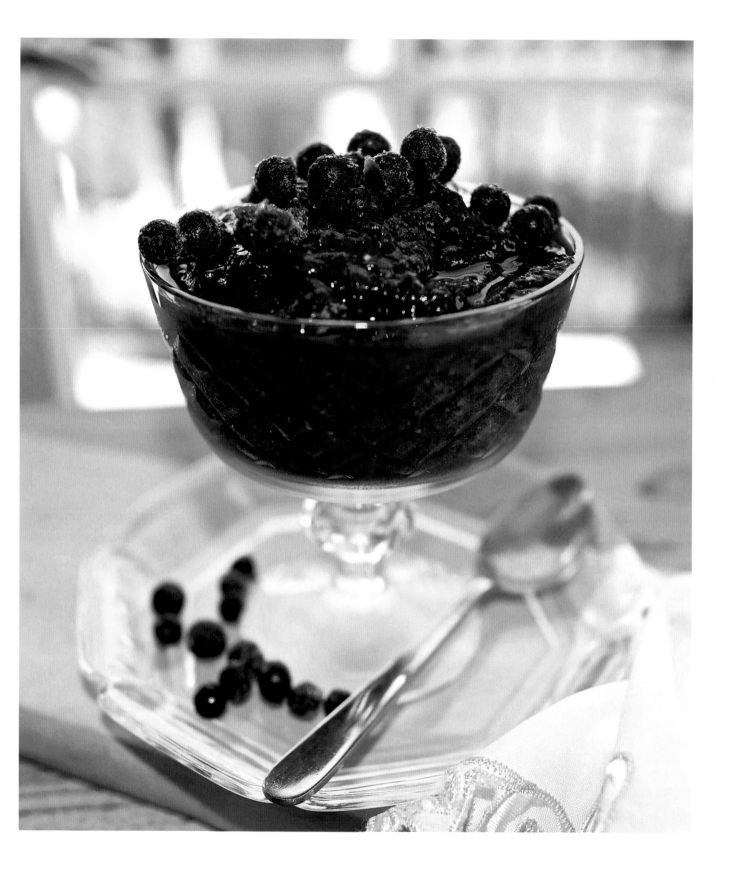

Quick Banana Walnut Breakfast

Mash banana with the milk in a cereal bowl. Add blueberries, walnut pieces, and ground flaxseeds and enjoy like a creamy bowl of cereal.

SERVES 1

1 banana

½ cup soy, hemp, or almond milk

½ cup blueberries or other berries

¼ cup walnut pieces

½ tablespoon ground flaxseeds

TIP: Remember the four high-omega-3 seeds and nuts: flaxseeds, chia and hemp seeds, and walnuts.

PER SERVING: CALORIES 377; PROTEIN 8g; CARBOHYDRATES 43g; TOTAL FAT 22.6g; SATURATED FAT 2.1g; SODIUM 97mg; FIBER 7.8g; BETA-CAROTENE 58mcg; VITAMIN C 18mg; CALCIUM 306mg; IRON 2.1mg; FOLATE 61mcg; MAGNESIUM 105mg; ZINC 1.4mg; SELENIUM 3.6mcg

Fruity Chickpea Cereal

SERVES 2

1 ½ cups cooked or 1 (15-ounce) can low-sodium or no-salt-added chickpeas, drained

2 bananas, sliced

Divide the chickpeas between two cereal bowls. Place bananas on top of beans. Refrigerate for about 5 minutes to chill.

Add berries or other fruit if desired.

PER SERVING: CALORIES 262; PROTEIN 9g; CARBOHYDRATES 53g; TOTAL FAT 3.2g; SATURATED FAT 0.4g; SODIUM 243mg; FIBER 3.1g; BETA-CAROTENE 46mcg; VITAMIN C 10mg; CALCIUM 55mg; IRON 1.4mg; FOLATE 70mcg; MAGNESIUM 59mg; ZINC 0.8mg; SELENIUM 1.2mcg

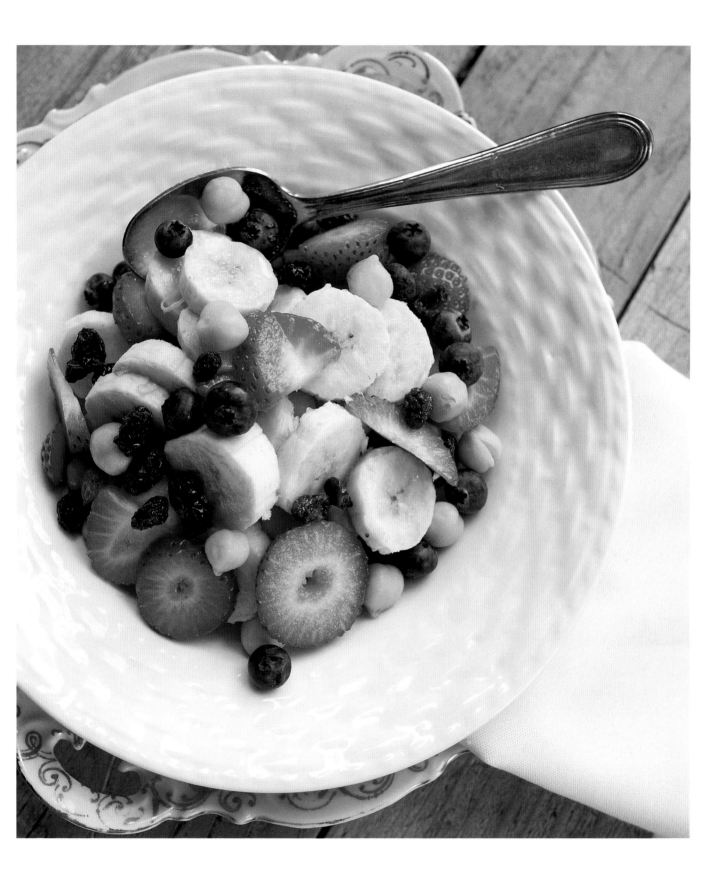

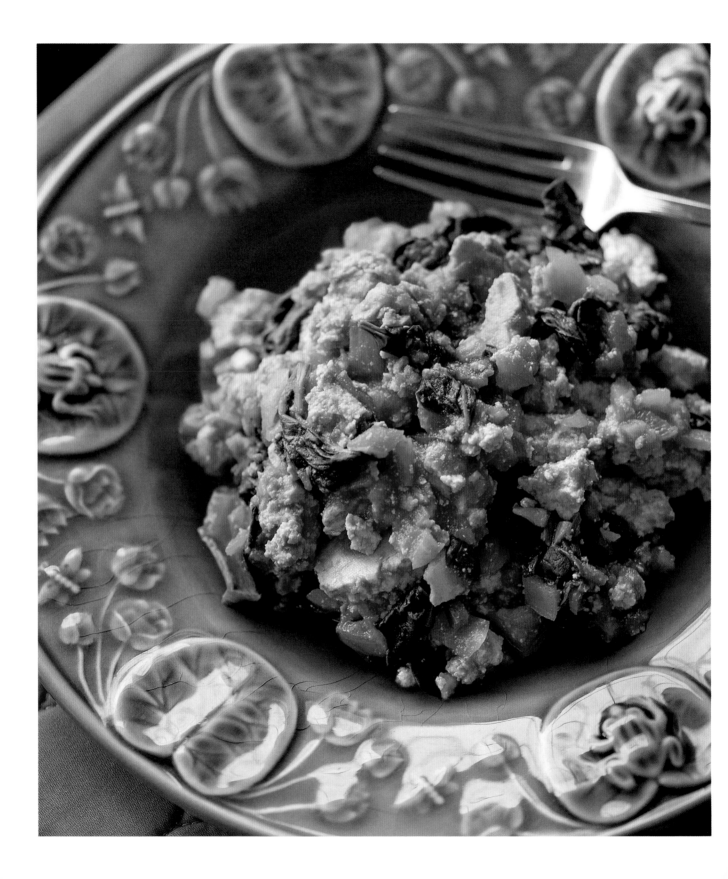

Tofu Scramble with Tomatoes and Peppers

Heat 2–3 tablespoons water in a large skillet and water-sauté peppers, onion, and garlic until tender. Add remaining ingredients and cook for another 5 minutes.

SERVES 2

1 cup chopped green, red, or yellow bell pepper

½ cup chopped onion

1 clove garlic, chopped

15 ounces (1 ½ cups) low-sodium diced tomatoes, drained*

14 ounces extra firm tofu, drained and crumbled

1 cup firmly packed spinach

1 teaspoon garlic powder

½ teaspoon turmeric (will turn tofu yellow like eggs)

¼ teaspoon red pepper flakes or ⅛ teaspoon chipotle powder, or to taste (optional)

Choose tomato products packed in cartons or glass rather than cans. These materials do not contain BPA.

PER SERVING: CALORIES 247; PROTEIN 21g; CARBOHYDRATES 20g; TOTAL FAT 9.8g; SATURATED FAT 1.3g; SODIUM 76mg; FIBER 6.2g; BETA-CAROTENE 2,182mcg; VITAMIN C 104mg; CALCIUM 398mg; IRON 4.9mg; FOLATE 79mcg; MAGNESIUM 42mg; ZINC 0.6mg; SELENIUM 1mcg

Creamy Breakfast Broccoli

SERVES 2

1 large head broccoli
(florets and stems)

1 leek

1 medium avocado, peeled,
pitted, and diced

Black pepper to taste

Steam broccoli florets and stems and the leek in a steamer until everything is soft enough to blend.

Process broccoli, leek, and diced avocado in a blender or food processor until creamy. Season with black pepper.

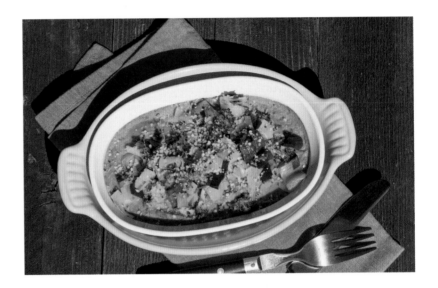

PER SERVING: CALORIES 244; PROTEIN 11g; CARBOHYDRATES 32g; TOTAL FAT 11.7g; SATURATED FAT 1.6g; SODIUM 115mg; FIBER 13.4g; BETA-CAROTENE 1,586mcg; VITAMIN C 282mg; CALCIUM 178mg; IRON 3.6mg; FOLATE 281mcg; MAGNESIUM 96mg; ZINC 1.8mg; SELENIUM 8.3mcg

SMOOTHIES AND BEVERAGES

Flood your cells with nutrients.

Smoothies are portable and require minimal time and effort to make. They are a great choice for on-the-run breakfasts or too-busy-to-eat lunches. And there's an added bonus: Blending fruits and raw, leafy vegetables makes it easier for the body to absorb the beneficial phytochemicals inside each plant's cells.

Keep a variety of frozen fruits and vegetables on hand so you are always ready to blend up a refreshing and healthy smoothie. Frozen produce is picked ripe and flash-frozen right on or near the farm, so its nutrient value is comparable to that of fresh. If you like your smoothie chilled, adding frozen fruit or a handful of ice cubes will do the trick.

Throw in a tablespoon of chia seeds, hemp seeds, or flaxseeds to make your smoothie even more nutritious. Unsweetened, natural cocoa powder is also a nice addition. It provides all the benefits and flavor of dark chocolate, with less fat and no added sugar. Of all chocolate products, cocoa powder has the highest concentration of flavanols—unique phytonutrients that have been shown to support healthy circulation and blood flow. Because Dutch processing or alkalizing reduces these naturally occurring compounds, choose a natural, nonalkalized cocoa. When choosing the greens, limit the amount of spinach you use to less than one-third of your raw vegetable intake because it is high in oxalic acid, which can interfere with calcium absorption.

Hot Oatmeal Smoothie

It doesn't take a lot of time to get your day off to a good start. Add oatmeal to your smoothie and blend for a few extra minutes to create a warm and satisfying breakfast.

Add ingredients to a high-powered blender. Gradually increase speed to high and run for 2–4 minutes, just until the mixture is warm. If blending is not warming sufficiently, microwave for one minute.

SERVES 1

½ cup unsweetened soy, hemp, or almond milk

2 tablespoons old-fashioned oats

1 cup strawberries, blueberries, or other fresh or frozen fruit

½ ounce walnuts (7 halves)

1 tablespoon raisins

¼ teaspoon cinnamon

½ tablespoon of flaxseeds

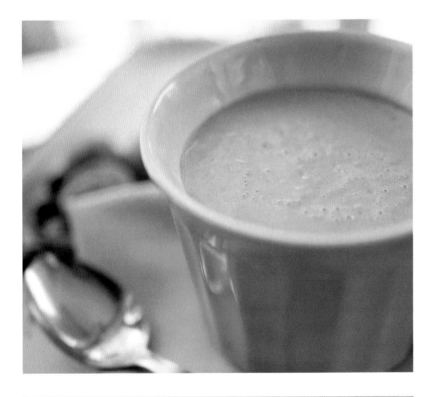

PER SERVING: CALORIES 279; PROTEIN 9g; CARBOHYDRATES 38g; TOTAL FAT 12.6g; SATURATED FAT 1.3g; SODIUM 49mg; FIBER 6.9g; BETA-CAROTENE 14mcg; VITAMIN C 98mg; CALCIUM 209mg; IRON 4.5mg; FOLATE 55mcg; MAGNESIUM 70mg; ZINC 1.2mg; SELENIUM 1.5mcg

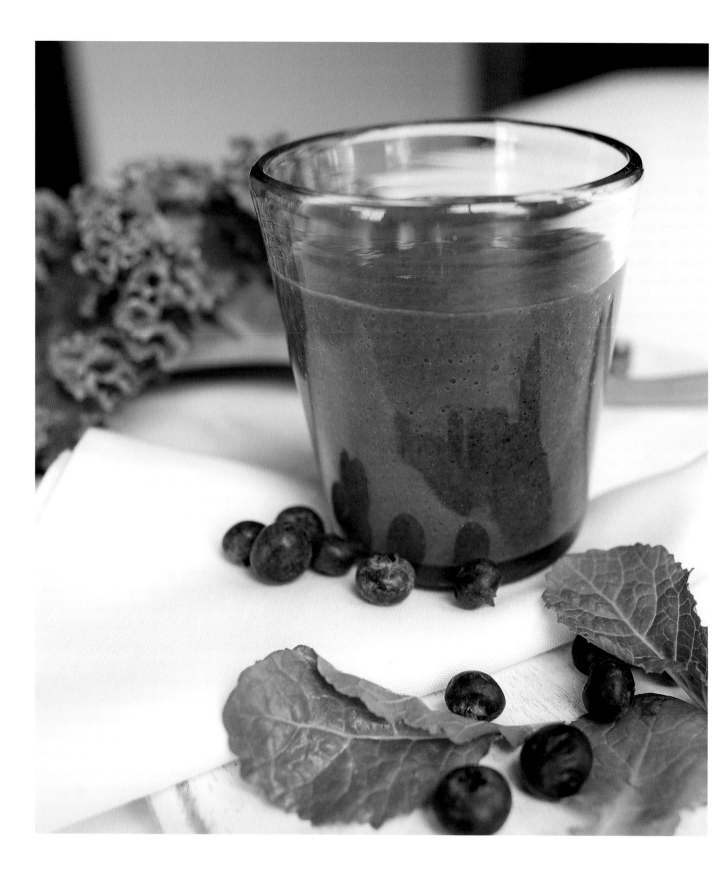

Go-To Green Smoothie

Get your cancer-fighting phytonutrients first thing in the morning with this trifecta of kale, seeds, and fruit polyphenols, and then go live life confidently.

Blend all ingredients in a high-powered blender.

3 cups chopped kale

½ banana*

1 cup fresh or frozen blueberries, strawberries, or cherries

¼ cup pomegranate juice or carrot juice

½ cup soy, hemp, or almond milk

1 tablespoon ground flaxseeds or chia seeds

* Freeze the other half of the banana to use for another smoothie or in one of the healthy ice cream recipes.

PER SERVING: CALORIES 334; PROTEIN 10g; CARBOHYDRATES 65g; TOTAL FAT 7.3g; SATURATED FAT 0.7g; SODIUM 188mg; FIBER 13.2g; BETA-CAROTENE 18,603mcg; VITAMIN C 250mg; CALCIUM 615mg; IRON 5.1mg; FOLATE 97mcg; MAGNESIUM 139mg; ZINC 1.7mg; SELENIUM 8mcg

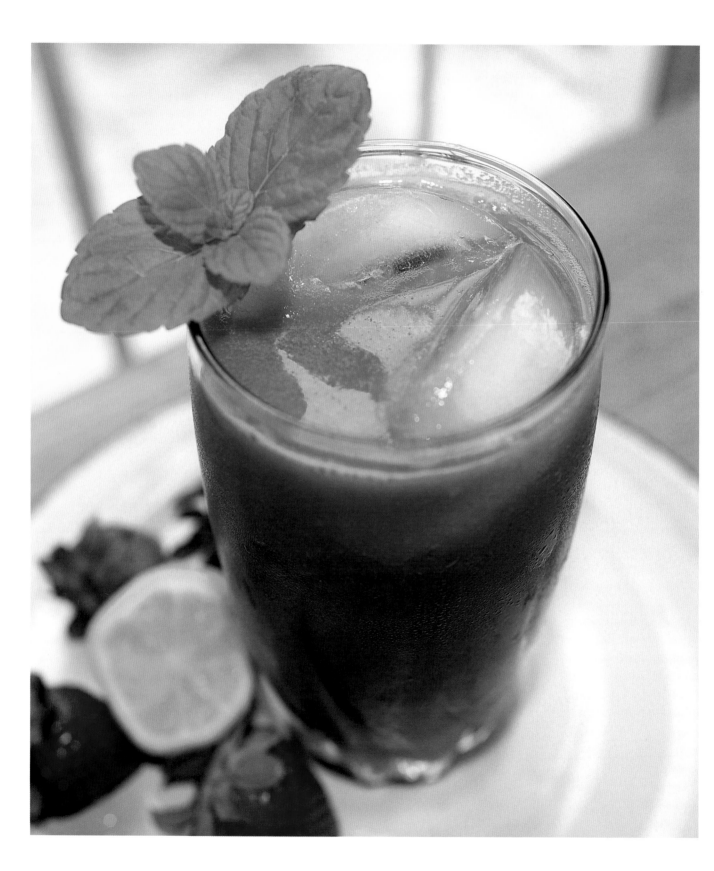

Green Lemonade

You have to taste this lemonade to believe that the healthiest lemonade in the world can taste out of this world.

Blend all ingredients in a high-powered blender.

SERVES 2

1 orange, peeled and seeded

2 lemons, juiced

2–3 dates, pitted

1 apple, peeled and cored

1 small piece fresh ginger, peeled

2–4 leaves kale

1 cup ice cubes

PER SERVING: CALORIES 122; PROTEIN 2g; CARBOHYDRATES 31g; TOTAL FAT 0.6g; SATURATED FAT 0.1g; SODIUM 21mg; FIBER 4g; BETA-CAROTENE 3,345mcg; VITAMIN C 106mg; CALCIUM 91mg; IRON 0.9mg; FOLATE 45mcg; MAGNESIUM 31mg; ZINC 0.3mg; SELENIUM 0.6mcg

Super-Easy Blended Salad

SERVES 1

8 ounces baby greens

1 orange, peeled and seeded

¼ lemon, juiced

Baby raw greens are super foods with a huge antioxidant content. Eat your greens every day.

Blend ingredients in a high-powered blender until smooth and creamy.

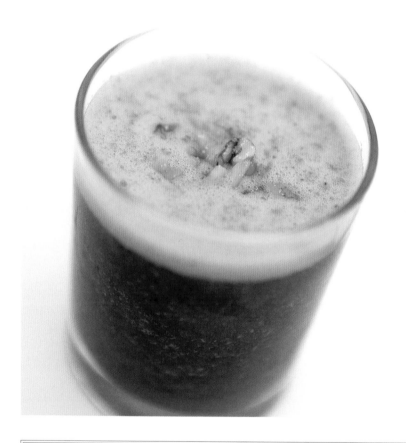

PER SERVING: CALORIES 119; PROTEIN 6g; CARBOHYDRATES 26g; TOTAL FAT 1.2g; SATURATED FAT 0.2g; SODIUM 57mg; FIBER 8.4g; BETA-CAROTENE 3,211mcg; VITAMIN C 112mg; CALCIUM 301mg; IRON 2.8mg; FOLATE 321mcg; MAGNESIUM 86mg; ZINC 1.5mg; SELENIUM 0.6mcg

Chocolate Peanut Butter Smoothie

This smoothie makes a great breakfast for kids of all ages.

Blend all ingredients in a blender.

Adjust the amount of nondairy milk to desired consistency. For added sweetness, add 1–2 pitted dates.

SERVES 1

2 cups baby kale

1 tablespoon natural, no-salt-added peanut butter

1 tablespoon natural cocoa powder

½ ripe frozen banana

½–1 cup soy, hemp, or almond milk

¼ teaspoon alcohol-free vanilla extract

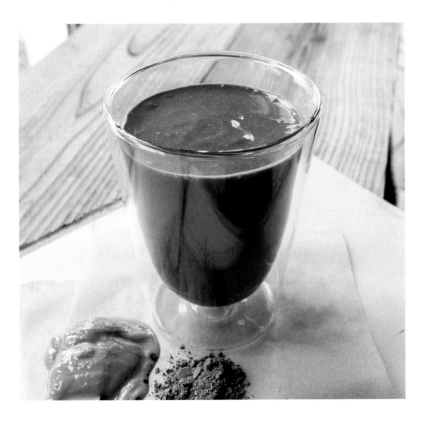

PER SERVING: CALORIES 285; PROTEIN 15g; CARBOHYDRATES 33g; TOTAL FAT 13.5g; SATURATED FAT 2.7g; SODIUM 132mg; FIBER 7g; BETA-CAROTENE 7,862mcg; VITAMIN C 107mg; CALCIUM 437mg; IRON 3.9mg; FOLATE 50mcg; MAGNESIUM 135mg; ZINC 2.3mg; SELENIUM 3mcg

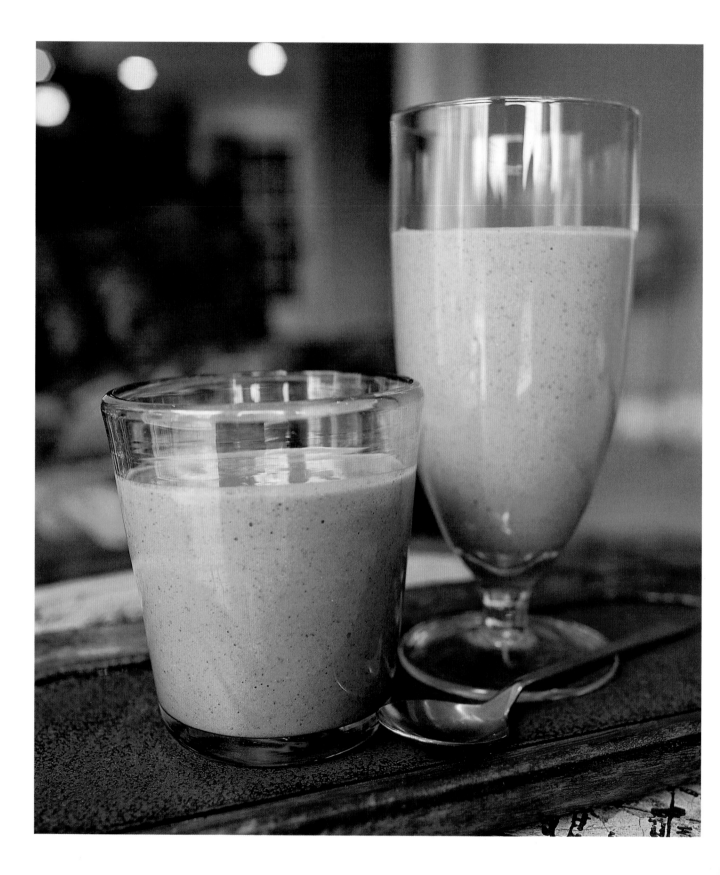

Chocolate Almond Smoothie

The whole is greater than the sum of its parts—polyphenols from cocoa mixed with greens, seeds, and nuts means that brain-protective phytochemicals are being more efficiently absorbed and utilized.

Blend all ingredients together in a high-powered blender until smooth and creamy.

1 cup kale

2 cups chopped romaine lettuce

2 tablespoons raw almond butter

2 tablespoons natural (nonalkalized) cocoa powder

1 ripe banana

1 cup soy, hemp, or almond milk

1 tablespoon ground flaxseeds

2 medjool dates or 4 regular dates, pitted

PER SERVING: CALORIES 313; PROTEIN 11g; CARBOHYDRATES 46g; TOTAL FAT 13.7g; SATURATED FAT 1.6g; SODIUM 68mg; FIBER 9.8g; BETA-CAROTENE 5,584mcg; VITAMIN C 47mg; CALCIUM 304mg; IRON 3.5mg; FOLATE 102mcg; MAGNESIUM 152mg; ZINC 2mg; SELENIUM 3.1mcg

Margarita Cooler

SERVES 4

3 cups green seedless grapes

1 lime, peeled and seeds removed

1 orange, peeled and seeds removed

6 ounces kale, large stems removed

Don't let the mild taste of kale fool you. It is a powerhouse of micro-nutrients and phytochemicals with dramatic health benefits. Why not enjoy drinks that protect your brain and make you smarter, rather than unhealthful drinks that can damage the brain?

Add ingredients to a high-powered blender and blend until smooth. Pour over ice.

PER SERVING: CALORIES 122; PROTEIN 3g; CARBOHYDRATES 31g; TOTAL FAT 0.6g; SATURATED FAT 0.1g; SODIUM 21mg; FIBER 3.1g; BETA-CAROTENE 4,003mcg; VITAMIN C 80mg; CALCIUM 89mg; IRON 1.3mg; FOLATE 28mcg; MAGNESIUM 27mg; ZINC 0.3mg; SELENIUM 0.6mcg

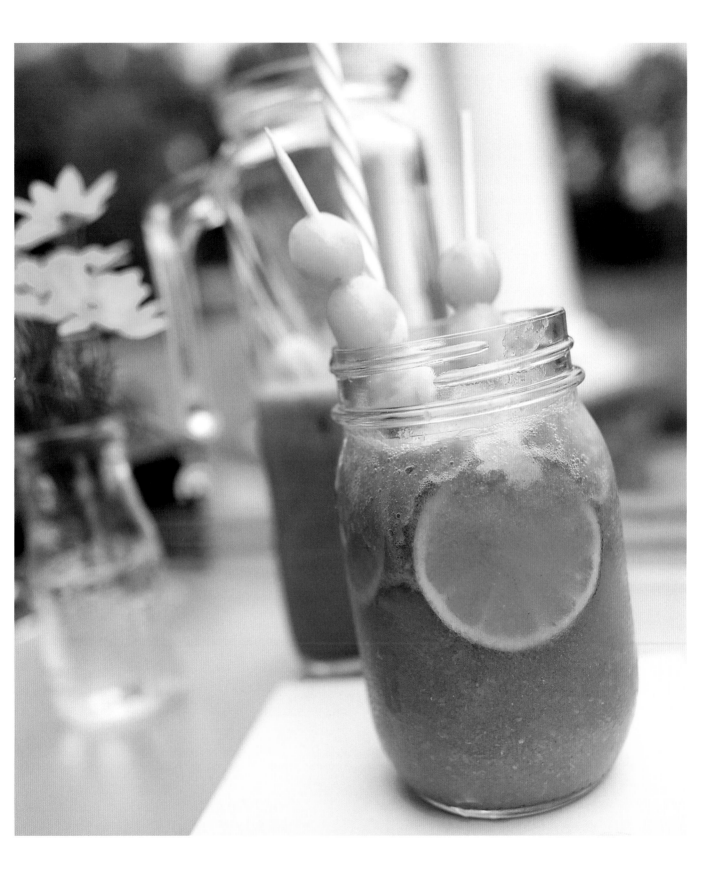

Orange Pomegranate Sparkler

SERVES 2

2 ounces pomegranate juice

1 orange, juiced*

1 tablespoon balsamic vinegar or other flavored vinegar

1 teaspoon lemon juice

1 cup seltzer water

4 ice cubes

....

If desired, you can substitute a peeled and seeded orange for the orange juice. Blend the orange with the pomegranate juice, vinegar, lemon juice, and ice. Pour into glasses and stir in the seltzer water.

Toast to good health with an elegant drink for your most prestigious event or have some as you luxuriate in the bathtub or lounge on the beach.

Combine ingredients and stir.

PER SERVING: CALORIES 48; PROTEIN 1g; CARBOHYDRATES 11g; TOTAL FAT 0.2g; SODIUM 10mg; FIBER 0.2g; BETA-CAROTENE 20mcg; VITAMIN C 32mg; CALCIUM 16mg; IRON 0.2mg; FOLATE 26mcg; MAGNESIUM 11mg; ZINC 0.1mg; SELENIUM 0.2mcg

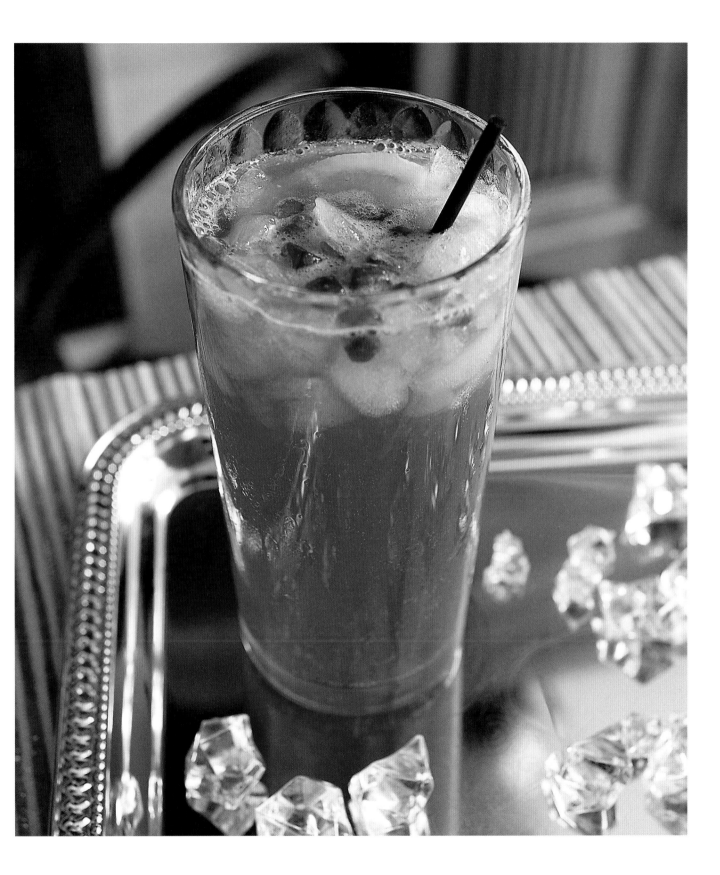

SALAD DRESSINGS

Make salad the main dish. It's the secret to successful weight control and a long, healthy life.

Instead of using low-nutrient, refined oils in your salad dressings, use real foods such as almonds and other nuts, sesame or other seeds, and avocado as the fat sources. Oils, even if they are monounsaturated, like olive oil, are not healthful—they are low in nutrients and contain 120 calories per tablespoon, which make them fattening.

Nut- and seed-based salad dressings ensure that we get the "good" fats we need, along with their antioxidants, phytochemicals, and other health-supporting benefits. The fat from nuts and seeds, when eaten with vegetables, increases the phytochemical absorption from those veggies.

Use unsalted, raw nuts and seeds. Commercial roasting can alter their beneficial fats. If you would like to lightly toast your raw nuts or seeds, arrange them in a single layer in a shallow roasting pan in a 300°F oven and roast 5–10 minutes, stirring and rotating occasionally until they are very lightly browned. Sesame seeds can be toasted on the stovetop in an ungreased skillet for 2–3 minutes, stirring frequently.

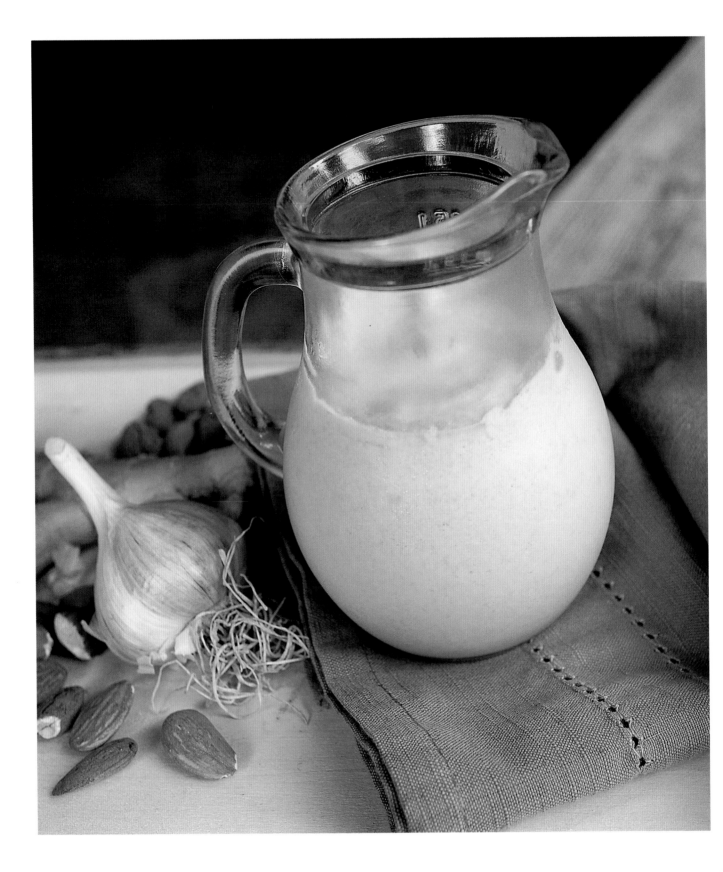

Ginger Almond Dressing

Blend all ingredients together in a high-powered blender until creamy. Add more nondairy milk if a thinner dressing is desired.

½ cup raw almonds or ¼ cup raw almond butter

2 tablespoons unhulled sesame seeds

½ cup unsweetened soy, hemp, or almond milk

2 tablespoons rice vinegar

3 regular dates or 1 ½ medjool dates, pitted

1 small clove garlic, chopped

½-inch piece fresh ginger, peeled and chopped

PER SERVING: CALORIES 217; PROTEIN 7g; CARBOHYDRATES 13g; TOTAL FAT 16.7g; SATURATED FAT 1.6g; SODIUM 18mg; FIBER 3.8g; BETA-CAROTENE 1mcg; VITAMIN C 1mg; CALCIUM 148mg; IRON 1.2mg; FOLATE 22mcg; MAGNESIUM 76mg; ZINC 1.3mg; SELENIUM 1mcg

Easy Balsamic Almond Dressing

SERVES 1

2 tablespoons water

1 tablespoon plus 1 teaspoon balsamic vinegar

1 tablespoon raw almond butter

¼ teaspoon onion powder

¼ teaspoon garlic powder

⅛ teaspoon dried oregano

⅛ teaspoon dried basil

Whisk water, vinegar, and almond butter together until mixture is smooth and almond butter is evenly dispersed.

Mix in remaining ingredients.

PER SERVING: CALORIES 127; PROTEIN 4g; CARBOHYDRATES 9g; TOTAL FAT 8.9g; SATURATED FAT 0.7g; SODIUM 10mg; FIBER 2g; BETA-CAROTENE 3mcg; CALCIUM 74mg; IRON 1.1mg; FOLATE 10mcg; MAGNESIUM 51mg; ZINC 0.6mg; SELENIUM 0.7mcg

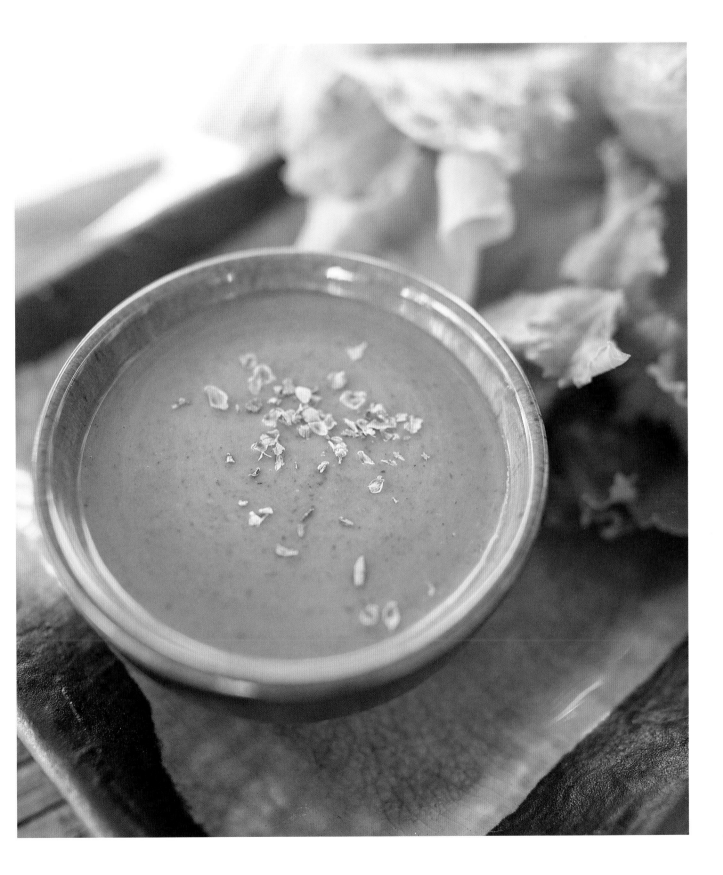

Banana Walnut Dressing

SERVES 2

2 bananas

2 tablespoons walnuts

2 tablespoons raisins

¼ cup fruit-flavored vinegar

Toss this dressing with mixed greens, create a kale salad, or use it as a dip for fresh fruit.

Blend all ingredients in a high-powered blender or food processor until smooth and creamy.

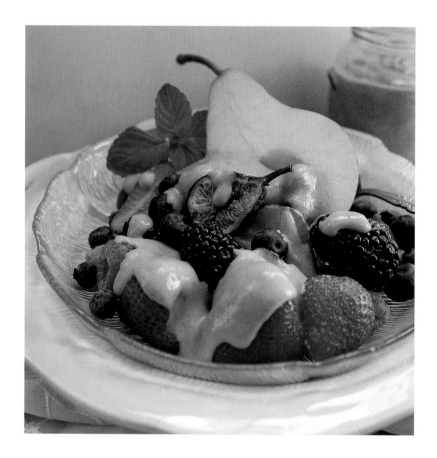

PER SERVING: CALORIES 163; PROTEIN 2g; CARBOHYDRATES 35g; TOTAL FAT 3g; SATURATED FAT 0.4g; SODIUM 3mg; FIBER 3.7g; BETA-CAROTENE 31mcg; VITAMIN C 11mg; CALCIUM 16mg; IRON 0.6mg; FOLATE 28mcg; MAGNESIUM 41mg; ZINC 0.3mg; SELENIUM 1.6mcg

Creamy Lemon Dressing

Put all ingredients in a high-powered blender and blend until very smooth.

SERVES 6

1 cup unsweetened soy, hemp, or almond milk

½ cup raw cashews

½ cup pecans

1 large lemon, juiced

2 teaspoons low-sodium mustard

2 cloves garlic, minced

½ cup flavored or balsamic vinegar

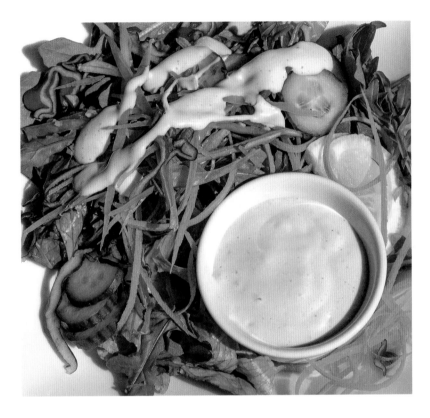

PER SERVING: CALORIES 151; PROTEIN 6g; CARBOHYDRATES 10g;
TOTAL FAT 10.8g; SATURATED FAT 1.9g; SODIUM 39mg; FIBER 1.4g;
BETA-CAROTENE 1mcg; VITAMIN C 8mg; CALCIUM 67mg; IRON 1.9mg;
FOLATE 7mcg; MAGNESIUM 76mg; ZINC 1.5mg; SELENIUM 5.3mcg

Orange Sesame Dressing

SERVES 4

2 oranges, peeled and seeded

¼ cup rice vinegar

¼ cup natural, no-salt-added peanut butter, or lightly roasted peanuts

1 teaspoon Bragg Liquid Aminos or low-sodium soy sauce

¼-inch piece fresh ginger, peeled

¼ clove garlic

Blend all ingredients in a high-powered blender until smooth.

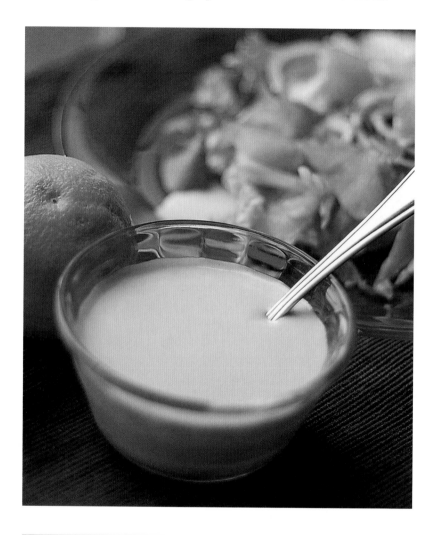

PER SERVING: CALORIES 133; PROTEIN 4g; CARBOHYDRATES 13g; TOTAL FAT 8.1g; SATURATED FAT 1.6g; SODIUM 59mg; FIBER 2.2g; BETA-CAROTENE 61mcg; VITAMIN C 41mg; CALCIUM 39mg; IRON 0.7mg; FOLATE 35mcg; MAGNESIUM 42mg; ZINC 0.7mg; SELENIUM 1.4mcg

Quick Avocado Dressing

The healthy fat in avocados helps you absorb more of the nutrients from the vegetables in your salad.

Blend all ingredients in a high-powered blender until smooth and creamy. You can modify the amounts of shallots and nondairy milk to adjust taste and consistency.

SERVES 4

2 ripe avocados, peeled, pitted, and chopped

2 tablespoons unfortified nutritional yeast

¼ cup unsweetened soy, hemp, or almond milk

2–3 small shallots, or to taste

¼ cup white wine vinegar

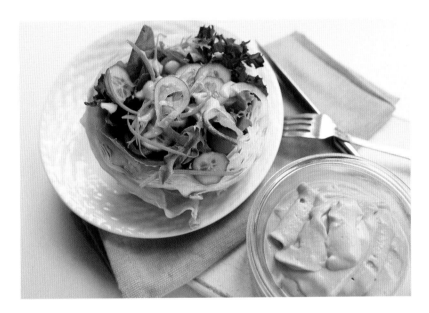

TIP: Unlike most fruits, avocados start to ripen only after they are picked. Unripe, firm, and green fruit can take four to five days to ripen. A ripe avocado yields to gentle pressure but is still firm. If your avocado is ripe before you are ready to eat it, you can refrigerate it to slow down the ripening process.

PER SERVING: CALORIES 143; PROTEIN 4g; CARBOHYDRATES 9g; TOTAL FAT 10.9g; SATURATED FAT 1.5g; SODIUM 14mg; FIBER 5.8g; BETA-CAROTENE 43mcg; VITAMIN C 7mg; CALCIUM 35mg; IRON 0.8mg; FOLATE 64mcg; MAGNESIUM 30mg; ZINC 1.4mg; SELENIUM 0.5mcg

Simple Vinaigrette

SERVES 8 (1½ CUPS)

½ cup flavored vinegar, such as
passion fruit or blood orange
vinegar

1 cup water

2 teaspoons arrowroot powder,
dissolved in an additional ¼ cup
cold water

Bring the vinegar and the cup of water to a boil in a small saucepan. Once boiling, whisk in the arrowroot–cold water mixture and let boil for 2 minutes, but no longer, whisking occasionally.

Remove from the heat and let cool to room temperature.

Refrigerate until ready to use.

PER SERVING: CALORIES 6; PROTEIN 0g; CARBOHYDRATES 1g; TOTAL FAT 0g; SATURATED FAT 0g; SODIUM 2mg; FIBER 0g; BETA-CAROTENE 0mcg; VITAMIN C 0mg; CALCIUM 2mg; IRON 0mg; FOLATE 0mcg; MAGNESIUM 1mg; ZINC 0mg; SELENIUM 0mcg

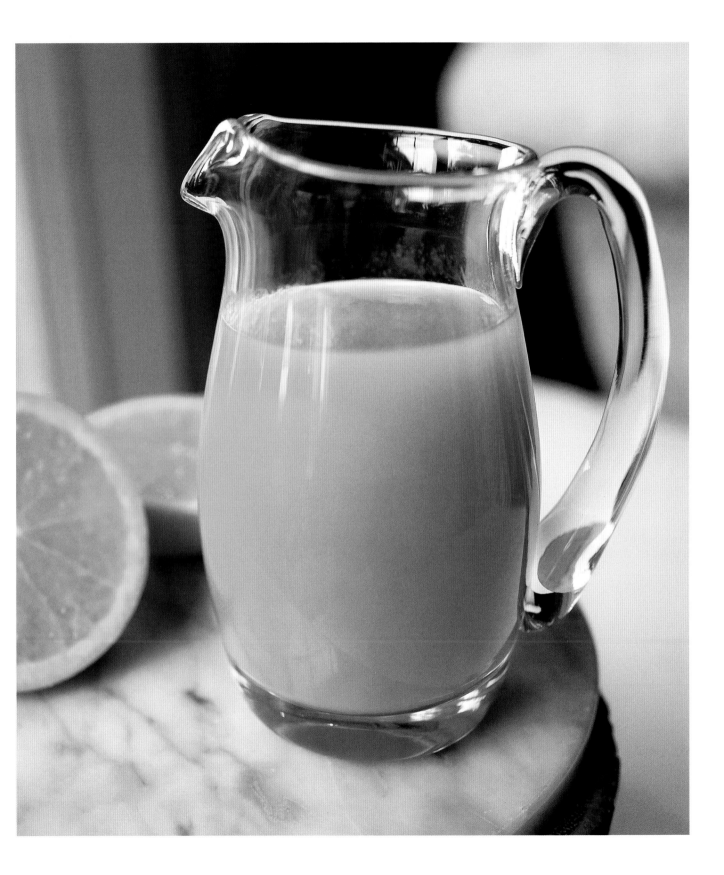

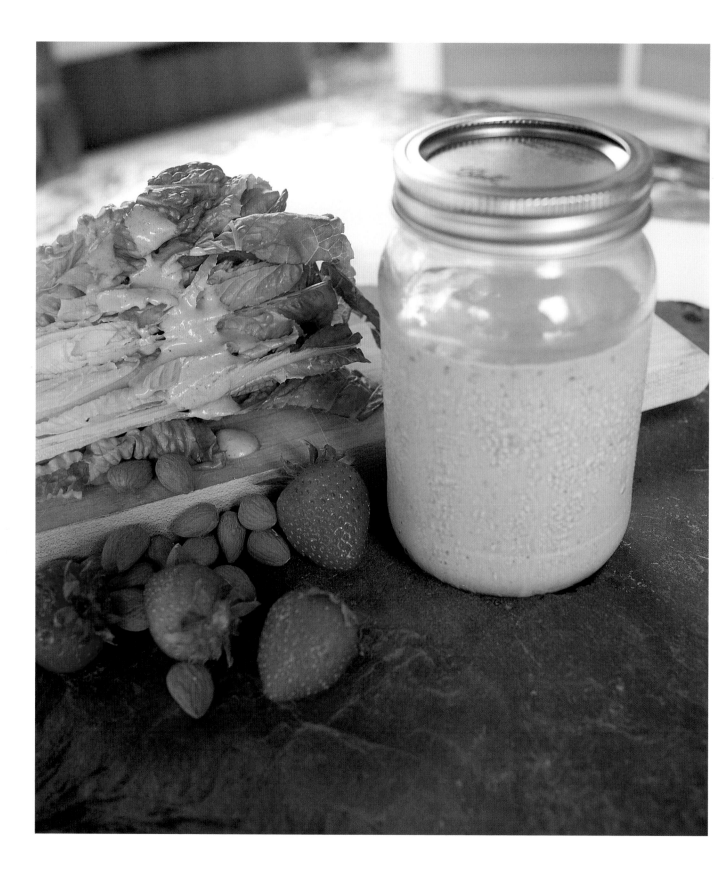

Strawberry Balsamic Dressing

Drain the almonds, reserving the soaking liquid.

Blend all ingredients in a high-powered blender until creamy, adding some of the soaking liquid to facilitate blending, until desired consistency is reached.

½ cup raw almonds, soaked overnight in water

½ pound fresh organic strawberries, hulled (or thawed frozen strawberries)

2 tablespoons balsamic vinegar

1 teaspoon almond extract

(Add 1 tablespoon raisins if strawberries are not very sweet)

PER SERVING: CALORIES 66; PROTEIN 2g; CARBOHYDRATES 5g; TOTAL FAT 4.4g; SATURATED FAT 0.3g; SODIUM 2mg; FIBER 1.7g; BETA-CAROTENE 8mcg; VITAMIN C 12mg; CALCIUM 29mg; IRON 0.6mg; FOLATE 9mcg; MAGNESIUM 28mg; ZINC 0.3mg; SELENIUM 0.4mcg

Ultimate Veggie Dressing

SERVES 4

1 cup leftover vegetable soup

½ cup raw cashews and/or pecans

2 tablespoons spicy pecan vinegar or other flavored vinegar

2 tablespoons unfortified nutritional yeast

Blend all ingredients in a blender.

PER SERVING: CALORIES 187; PROTEIN 6g; CARBOHYDRATES 26g; TOTAL FAT 9g; SATURATED FAT 1.2g; SODIUM 18mg; FIBER 2.1g; BETA-CAROTENE 83mcg; VITAMIN C 11mg; CALCIUM 26mg; IRON 1.5mg; FOLATE 11mcg; MAGNESIUM 48mg; ZINC 1.7mg; SELENIUM 2.7mcg

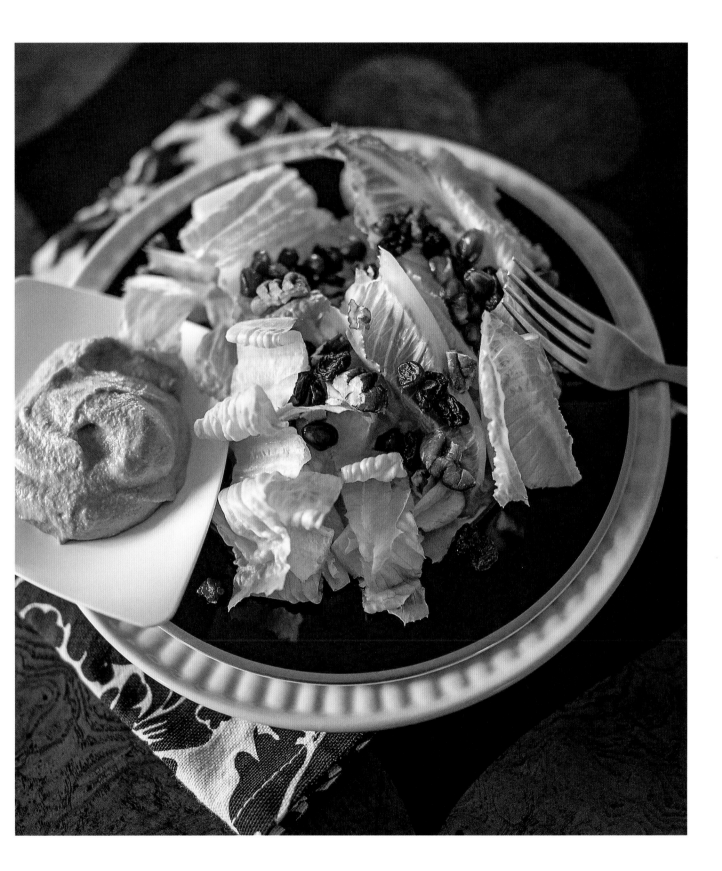

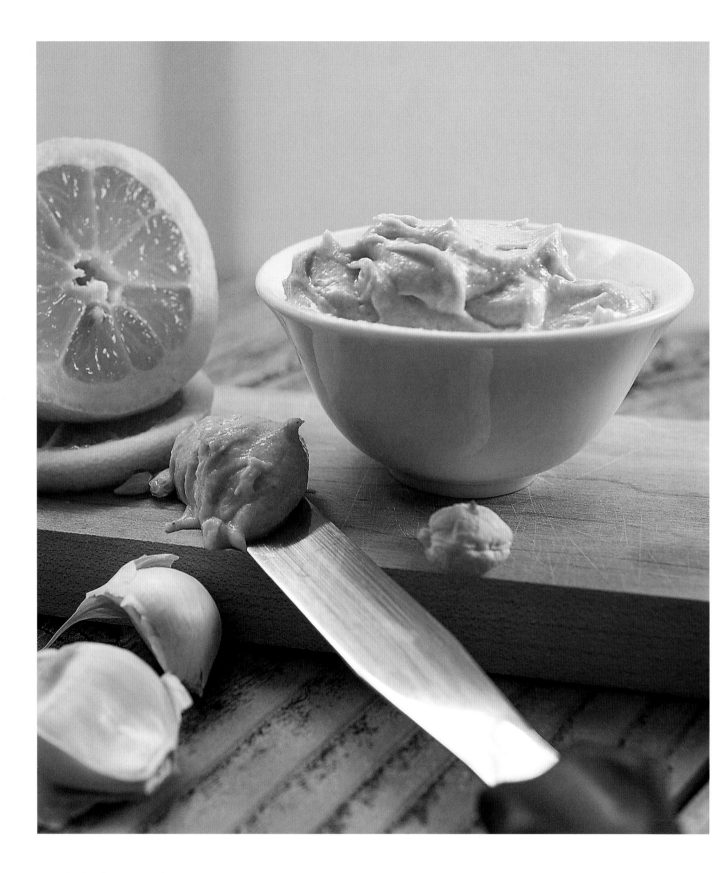

Better-for-You "Mayo"

Try this yummy spread on bean burgers or veggie wraps, or as salad dressing or dip.

Looking for something even quicker and easier? Nuttynaise Spread and Dressing, a nut- and seed-based mayonnaise substitute, is available at www.drfuhrman.com/shop.

Blend all ingredients together in a high-powered blender until creamy.

SERVES 5

1 cup raw cashews, soaked in water for 2 hours, then drained

3 regular dates or 1 ½ medjool dates, pitted

2 cloves garlic

2 tablespoons apple cider vinegar

½ lemon, juiced

PER SERVING: CALORIES 160; PROTEIN 5g; CARBOHYDRATES 12g; TOTAL FAT 11.4g; SATURATED FAT 2g; SODIUM 4mg; FIBER 1.2g; VITAMIN C 2mg; CALCIUM 14mg; IRON 1.8mg; FOLATE 8mcg; MAGNESIUM 79mg; ZINC 1.5mg; SELENIUM 5.5mcg

SALADS

When it comes to salads, think big!

The Standard American Diet (SAD) consists of 54 percent processed foods and 32 percent animal products. It contains only a small amount of greens, mushrooms, onions, seeds, colorful vegetables, and fruits. This leads to overall deficiencies in micronutrients, especially the antioxidants and phytochemicals necessary for normal health, cellular repair, and immune system function.

Make salad your main dish. Enjoy large salads composed of a variety of greens and other vegetables, including tomatoes, sliced onion, shredded cabbage, and lightly sautéed mushrooms. (As a safety precaution, I recommend cooking mushrooms because it significantly reduces potentially harmful compounds that are found in raw mushrooms.)

Experiment with lots of different ingredients and dressings. These easy recipes offer some creative combinations that work for many different occasions.

Fruity Salads

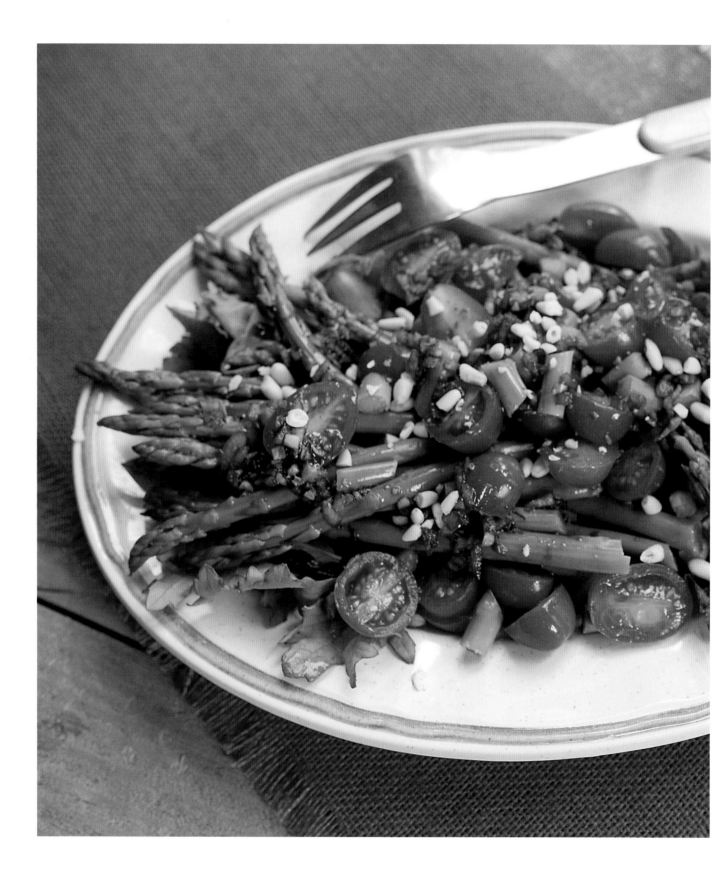

Balsamic Tomato and Asparagus Salad

Steam asparagus until just tender, about 12 minutes. Rinse with cold water to stop cooking, then drain. Mix with tomatoes.

Combine vinegar, orange juice, red onion, and black pepper. Add to asparagus and tomatoes and toss to coat. Refrigerate for at least 15 minutes so flavors can blend.

Serve on a bed of baby greens. Sprinkle with pine nuts before serving.

SERVES 4

1 pound asparagus, tough ends removed, cut into 2-inch pieces

1 cup cherry or grape tomatoes, cut in half

2 tablespoons balsamic vinegar

1 tablespoon orange juice

2 tablespoons minced red onion

Black pepper to taste

5 ounces mixed baby greens

3 tablespoons pine nuts, half chopped and half left whole

PER SERVING: CALORIES 90; PROTEIN 5g; CARBOHYDRATES 10g; TOTAL FAT 4.7g; SATURATED FAT 0.4g; SODIUM 26mg; FIBER 4.1g; BETA-CAROTENE 2,059mcg; VITAMIN C 21mg; CALCIUM 64mg; IRON 3.6mg; FOLATE 130mcg; MAGNESIUM 57mg; ZINC 1.3mg; SELENIUM 2.9mcg

Black Bean and Avocado Salad

SERVES 4

1 ½ cups cooked or 1 (15-ounce) can no-salt-added or low-sodium black beans, drained and rinsed

3 plum tomatoes, diced

¾ cup thawed frozen corn

¼ cup diced red bell pepper

¼ cup diced red onion

2 tablespoons chopped cilantro

½ jalapeño pepper, diced and seeded

2 tablespoons red wine vinegar

½ lime, juiced

¼ teaspoon ground cumin

2 avocados

Avocado halves make creative and tasty serving bowls for this zesty black bean salad.

Mix all ingredients except avocados and refrigerate for 1 hour.

Cut the avocados in half and remove the pits. Scoop out about 2 tablespoons of avocado from each half and mix into salad. Fill the avocado baskets with the salad.

PER SERVING: CALORIES 243; PROTEIN 9g; CARBOHYDRATES 30g; TOTAL FAT 11.3g; SATURATED FAT 1.6g; SODIUM 15mg; FIBER 12g; BETA-CAROTENE 435mcg; VITAMIN C 30mg; CALCIUM 37mg; IRON 2.2mg; FOLATE 184mcg; MAGNESIUM 84mg; ZINC 1.5mg; SELENIUM 1.3mcg

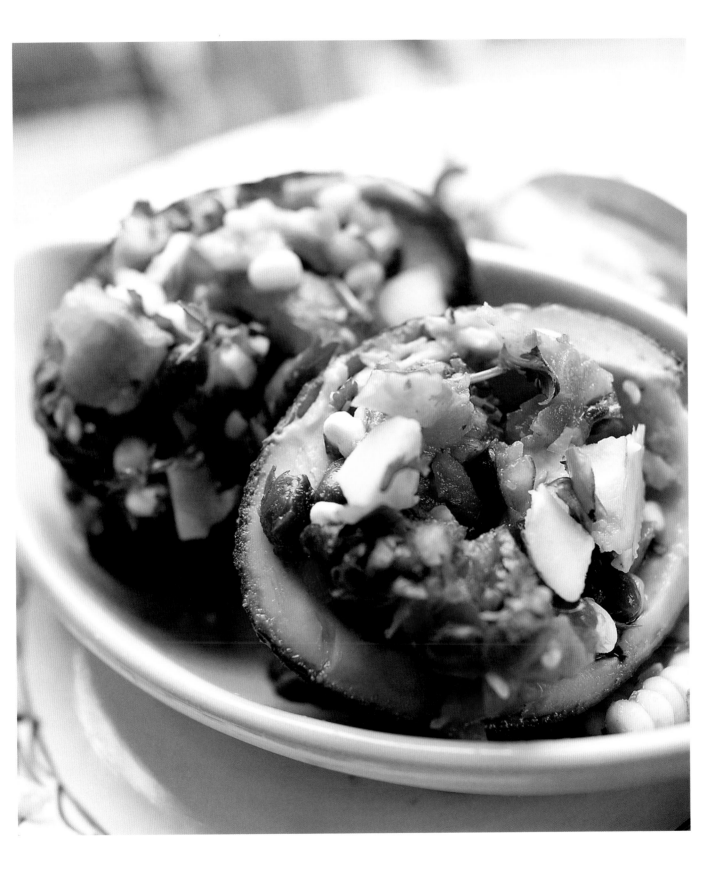

Broccoli Pomegranate Salad

SERVES 6

2 large heads broccoli, florets cut to bite size

¼ cup plus 2 tablespoons raisins, divided

¼ cup raw sunflower seeds

¼ cup chopped onion

¾ cup pomegranate juice

½ cup raw cashew butter

This super simple salad is ready in minutes and stores well in the refrigerator. It's perfect for lunch or a quick dinner side dish.

Combine broccoli, ¼ cup raisins, sunflower seeds, and onion in large bowl.

For dressing, combine pomegranate juice, remaining 2 tablespoons raisins, and cashew butter in a high-powered blender and blend until smooth, but not too thin.

Pour dressing over broccoli mixture and stir all together. Chill and serve.

PER SERVING: CALORIES 275; PROTEIN 11g; CARBOHYDRATES 32g; TOTAL FAT 14.4g; SATURATED FAT 2.5g; SODIUM 75mg; FIBER 6.7g; BETA-CAROTENE 733mcg; VITAMIN C 182mg; CALCIUM 118mg; IRON 3.1mg; FOLATE 165mcg; MAGNESIUM 122mg; ZINC 2.3mg; SELENIUM 10.8mcg

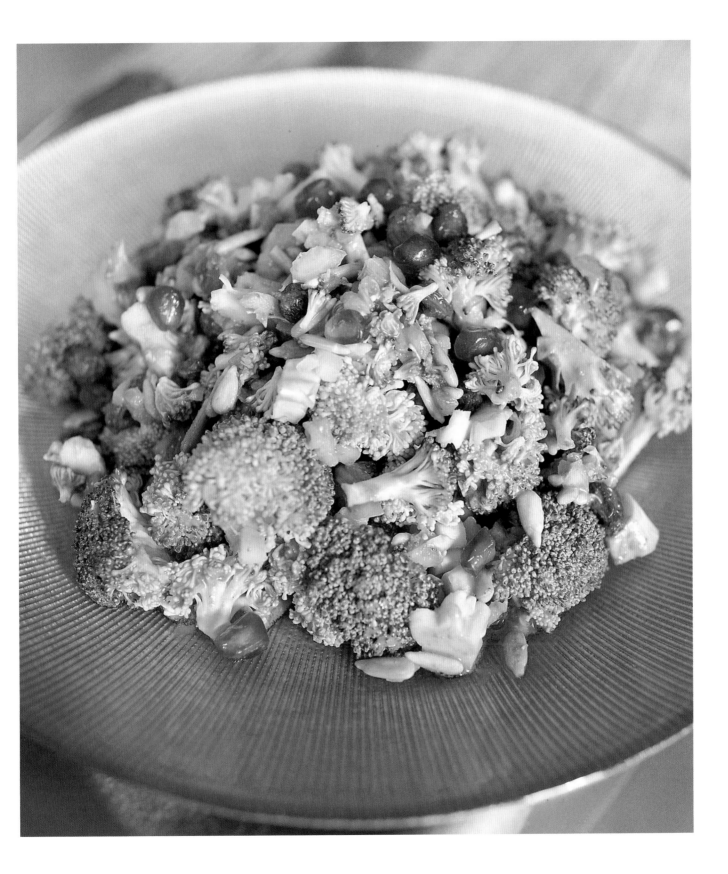

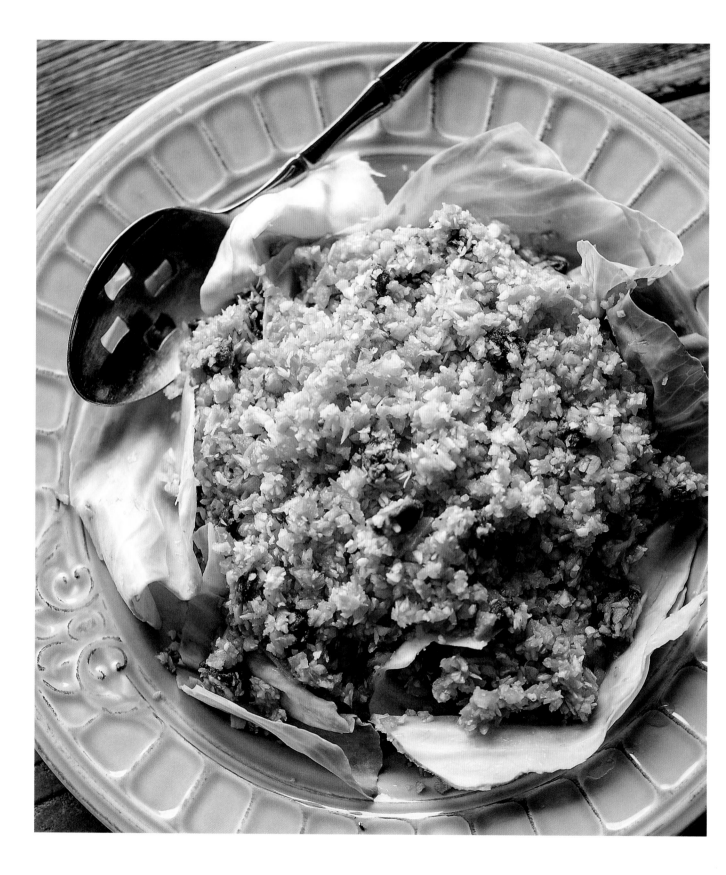

Sweet Shredded Carrot Salad

Combine carrots and raisins.

Add orange juice and cinnamon and mix all ingredients together.

SERVES 2

8 medium carrots, shredded*

½ cup raisins

4 tablespoons freshly squeezed orange juice

¼ teaspoon cinnamon, or to taste

* To save time, use a food processor to shred the carrots.

PER SERVING: CALORIES 209; PROTEIN 3g; CARBOHYDRATES 52g; TOTAL FAT 0.8g; SATURATED FAT 0.1g; SODIUM 172mg; FIBER 8.3g; BETA-CAROTENE 20,216mcg; VITAMIN C 15mg; CALCIUM 102mg; IRON 1.4mg; FOLATE 48mcg; MAGNESIUM 41mg; ZINC 0.7mg; SELENIUM 0.5mcg

Old-Fashioned Grain and Mushroom Salad

For the salad

1 cup uncooked farro

10 ounces mushrooms, sliced

¼ cup chopped red onion

3 cups baby arugula

For the dressing

1 medium tomato, quartered

⅓ cup raw cashews

¼ cup water

½ lime, juiced

1 tablespoon balsamic vinegar

In a saucepan, heat 2 cups water to boiling. Stir in farro; return to a boil. Reduce heat to low, then cover and cook for 20–25 minutes or until farro is tender. Drain.

Meanwhile, water-sauté mushrooms until they are soft and lightly browned. Combine cooked farro, mushrooms, chopped onion, and arugula.

Blend dressing ingredients together in a high-powered blender. Add desired amount of dressing to salad and toss. Serve warm or at room temperature.

TIP: Mushrooms activate superior immune function and strong protection against cancer. Even a small amount of mushrooms eaten daily shows this benefit. Keep a container of lightly sautéed mushrooms in your fridge so you can easily add them to salads and vegetable dishes.

PER SERVING: CALORIES 272; PROTEIN 11g; CARBOHYDRATES 42g; TOTAL FAT 7.7g; SATURATED FAT 1.2g; SODIUM 18mg; FIBER 5.0g; BETA-CAROTENE 213mcg; VITAMIN C 10mg; CALCIUM 66mg; IRON 3.4mg; FOLATE 109mcg; MAGNESIUM 137mg; ZINC 2.9mg; SELENIUM 24.7mcg

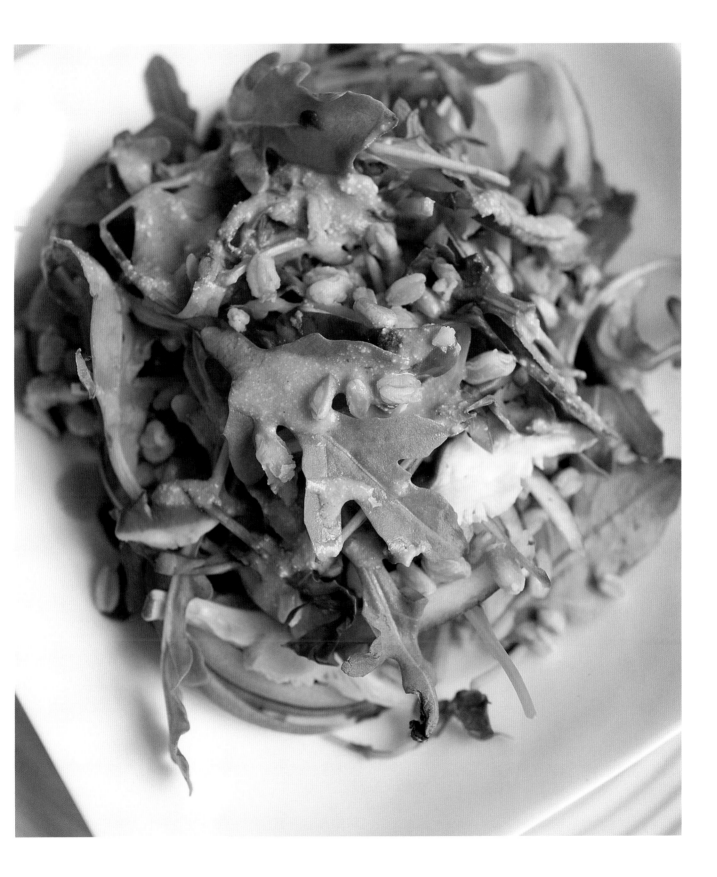

Green Bean Salad with Lemon Basil Vinaigrette

SERVES 6

For the salad

1 ½ pounds slender green beans, ends trimmed

1 cup cherry tomatoes, sliced in half

2 tablespoons chopped red onion

For the dressing

2 tablespoons balsamic vinegar

2 tablespoons fresh lemon juice

½ cup water

¼ cup plus 2 tablespoons raw almonds

¼ cup raisins

⅓ cup fresh basil leaves

1 teaspoon Dijon mustard

1 clove garlic

The Lemon Basil Vinaigrette also works well with a simple salad of mixed greens.

Steam green beans for 6 minutes or until crisp-tender. Transfer to a bowl and combine with tomatoes and red onion.

In a high-powered blender, blend the vinegar, lemon juice, water, ¼ cup almonds, raisins, basil, mustard, and garlic until smooth.

Toss bean mixture with desired amount of dressing. Chop remaining almonds and sprinkle on top.

PER SERVING: CALORIES 223; PROTEIN 10g; CARBOHYDRATES 37g; TOTAL FAT 4.9g; SATURATED FAT 0.4g; SODIUM 22mg; FIBER 12.5g; BETA-CAROTENE 195mcg; VITAMIN C 8mg; CALCIUM 106mg; IRON 1.9mg; FOLATE 96mcg; MAGNESIUM 93mg; ZINC 1.1mg; SELENIUM 2mcg

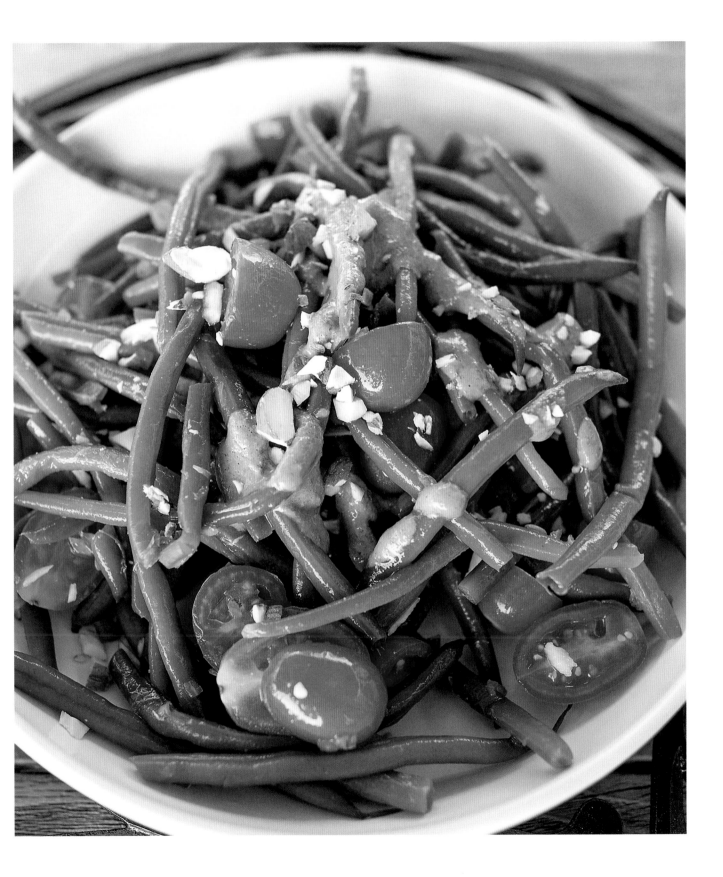

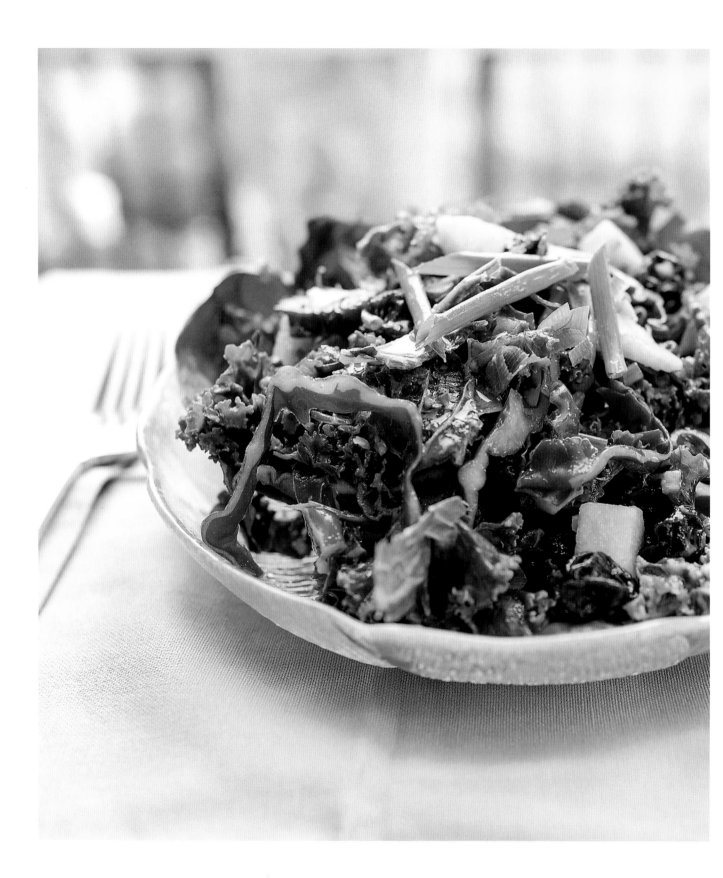

Kale and Red Cabbage Salad

Roll up each kale leaf and slice thinly. Place in a bowl along with avocado, lemon juice, and vinegar.

Using your hands, massage the avocado, lemon juice, and vinegar into the kale leaves until the kale starts to soften and wilt and each leaf is coated, about 2–3 minutes.

Mix in red cabbage, apple, dried fruit, and onion.

SERVES 2

1 bunch kale, tough stems and center ribs removed

1 avocado, peeled and chopped

2 tablespoons lemon juice

1 tablespoon white balsamic vinegar

1 cup thinly sliced red cabbage

1 large apple, cored and chopped

2 tablespoons raisins or unsweetened, unsulfured dried cherries

½ medium red onion, minced

PER SERVING: CALORIES 317; PROTEIN 8g; CARBOHYDRATES 53g; TOTAL FAT 12g; SATURATED FAT 1.7g; SODIUM 92mg; FIBER 12.4g; BETA-CAROTENE 15,840mcg; VITAMIN C 244mg; CALCIUM 270mg; IRON 3.9mg; FOLATE 130mcg; MAGNESIUM 94mg; ZINC 1.4mg; SELENIUM 2.2mcg

Peach and Leafy Lentil Salad

SERVES 4

For the salad

1 cup dry brown or green lentils, rinsed

4 cups water

1 head romaine lettuce, chopped

1 head red leaf lettuce, chopped

½ small red onion, finely chopped

2 cups ripe chopped peach, nectarine, or mango

For the dressing

½ cup freshly squeezed orange juice

2 tablespoons balsamic vinegar

¼ cup raw almonds

¼ cup raisins

1 clove garlic

Adding lentils and other beans to salads is genius. The body digests them slowly, which stabilizes blood sugar levels and reduces hunger and food cravings.

Bring lentils and water to a boil, cover, reduce heat, and simmer until lentils are tender but not mushy, about 20–25 minutes, stirring occasionally. Drain.

In a large mixing bowl, toss together the lettuce, red onion, fruit, and lentils.

To make dressing, blend remaining ingredients in a high-powered blender until smooth and creamy.

Toss salad with desired amount of dressing.

PER SERVING: CALORIES 326; PROTEIN 18g; CARBOHYDRATES 58g; TOTAL FAT 4.3g; SATURATED FAT 0.4g; SODIUM 51mg; FIBER 21.1g; BETA-CAROTENE 11,772mcg; VITAMIN C 27mg; CALCIUM 203mg; IRON 6.8mg; FOLATE 457mcg; MAGNESIUM 122mg; ZINC 3.2mg; SELENIUM 6.1mcg

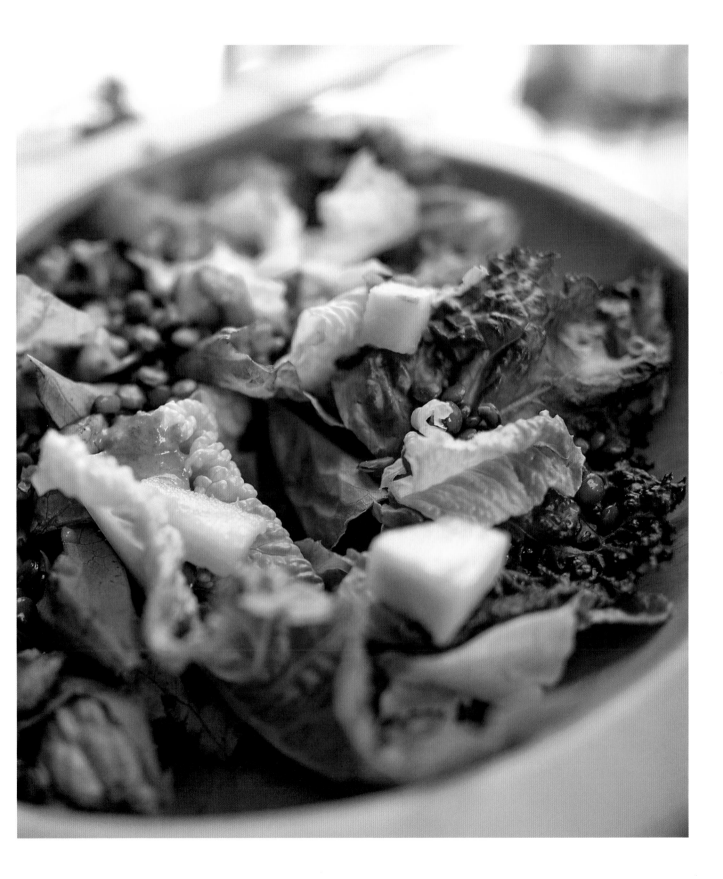

Quick and Easy Bean Salad

1 ½ cups cooked or 1 (15-ounce) can low-sodium or no-salt-added cannellini beans or other white beans, drained

½ small red onion, chopped

1 tomato, chopped

½ cup chopped parsley

1 tablespoon balsamic vinegar

1 teaspoon no-salt seasoning blend, adjusted to taste

Mix all the ingredients in a bowl.

Serve cold as a salad or heat in the microwave for a warm entrée.

PER SERVING: CALORIES 219; PROTEIN 14g; CARBOHYDRATES 40g; TOTAL FAT 0.8g; SATURATED FAT 0.2g; SODIUM 24mg; FIBER 10.8g; BETA-CAROTENE 963mcg; VITAMIN C 28mg; CALCIUM 157mg; IRON 6.3mg; FOLATE 147mcg; MAGNESIUM 103mg; ZINC 2.2mg; SELENIUM 1.9mcg

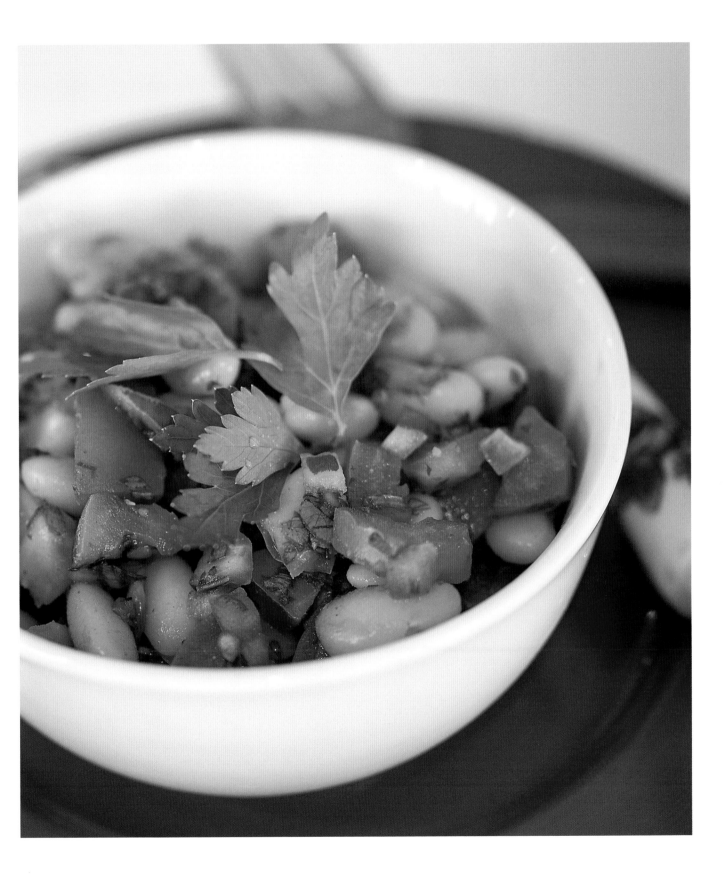

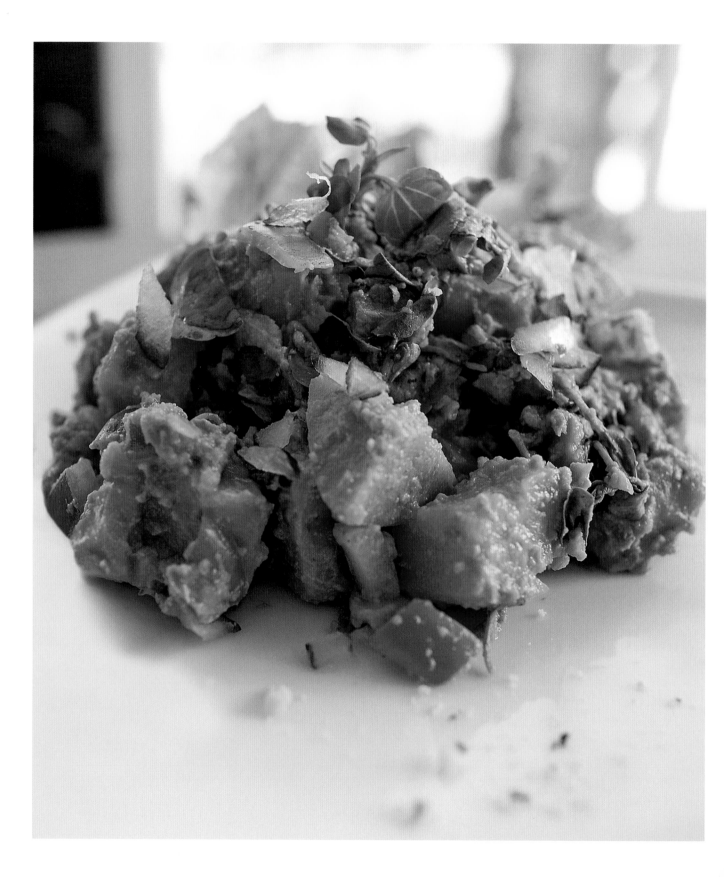

Sweet Potato Salad

Sweet potatoes and watercress make an unusual but winning combination in this different and delicious salad. Watercress is one of the most nutrient-dense green vegetables.

Add potatoes to a large pot of cold water. Bring to a boil over medium heat and cook until the potatoes are tender but not mushy, about 8–12 minutes. Drain.

Meanwhile, to prepare dressing, combine vinegar, water, walnuts, raisins, mustard, and garlic in a high-powered blender. Blend until smooth.

Place potatoes in a large bowl along with onion, red pepper, and watercress. Add desired amount of dressing and toss to combine. Season with black pepper. Serve warm or cold.

SERVES 6

6 medium sweet potatoes, peeled and cut into 1-inch pieces

¼ cup balsamic vinegar

½ cup water

¼ cup walnuts

¼ cup raisins

1 teaspoon Dijon mustard

1 clove garlic

½ medium red onion, finely chopped

1 red bell pepper, finely chopped

1 bunch watercress, large stems removed

Black pepper to taste

TIP: A nutrient-dense, plant-rich diet is effective for long-term weight control because you feel full and satisfied, even when consuming fewer calories.

PER SERVING: CALORIES 182; PROTEIN 4g; CARBOHYDRATES 35g; TOTAL FAT 3.4g; SATURATED FAT 0.3g; SODIUM 98mg; FIBER 5g; BETA-CAROTENE 11,766mcg; VITAMIN C 29mg; CALCIUM 89mg; IRON 1.3mg; FOLATE 28mcg; MAGNESIUM 52mg; ZINC 0.6mg; SELENIUM 1.7mcg

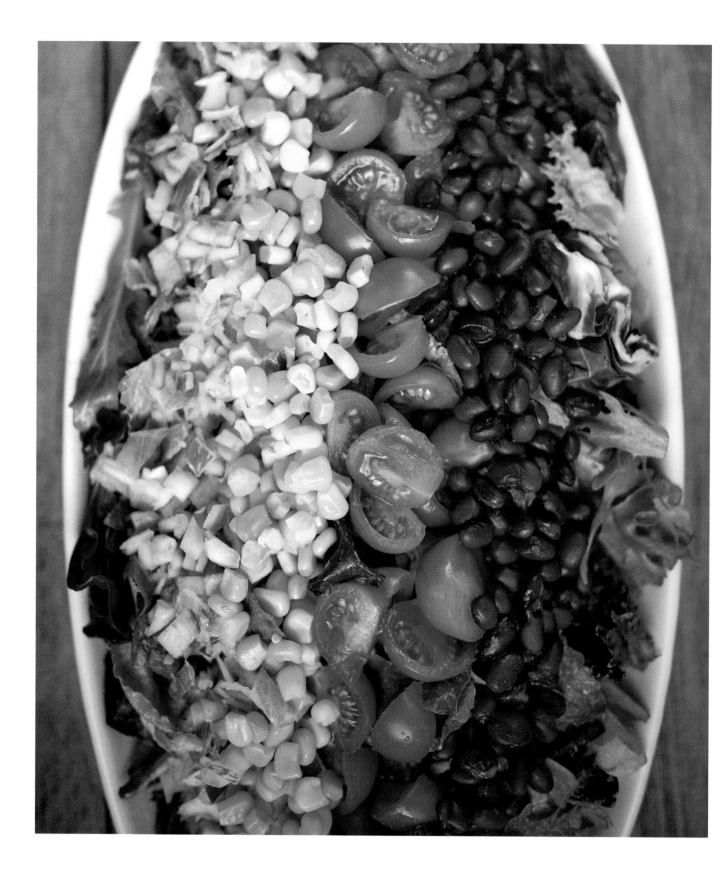

Tex-Mex Salad

Place dressing ingredients in a blender or food processor and blend until smooth.

Combine salad ingredients in a large bowl and toss with desired amount of dressing.

SERVES 2

For the dressing

1 ripe avocado, peeled and pit removed

½ lime, juiced

1 small clove garlic, chopped

1 tablespoon unfortified nutritional yeast

Pinch of cayenne pepper, or more to taste

For the salad

6 cups romaine lettuce, chopped

4 cups mixed baby greens

1 cup cooked black beans

1 cup thawed frozen corn kernels

1 medium tomato, chopped

¼ cup chopped red onion

PER SERVING: CALORIES 380; PROTEIN 17g; CARBOHYDRATES 59g; TOTAL FAT 12.5g; SATURATED FAT 1.8g; SODIUM 41mg; FIBER 20.2g; BETA-CAROTENE 10,236mcg; VITAMIN C 35mg; CALCIUM 121mg; IRON 5.3mg; FOLATE 427mcg; MAGNESIUM 148mg; ZINC 3.4mg; SELENIUM 3.7mcg

Kale and Fruit Salad with Almond Citrus Dressing

SERVES 2

For the dressing

¼ cup raw almonds

2 oranges, juiced

2 teaspoons balsamic vinegar

6 large chunks fresh pineapple

For the salad

4–6 leaves curly green kale, finely chopped

1 apple, chopped into chunks

1 cup red grapes, whole or sliced

1 cup fresh mango, in chunks

This yummy dressing works well with any combination of leafy greens.

Combine the dressing ingredients in a high-powered blender. Toss desired amount of dressing with the salad ingredients.

Refrigerate leftover dressing for another use.

PER SERVING: CALORIES 397; PROTEIN 11g; CARBOHYDRATES 74g; TOTAL FAT 11.3g; SATURATED FAT 1g; SODIUM 67mg; FIBER 9.9g; BETA-CAROTENE 12,995mcg; VITAMIN C 268mg; CALCIUM 265mg; IRON 3.8mg; FOLATE 121mcg; MAGNESIUM 130mg; ZINC 1.4mg; SELENIUM 2.5mcg

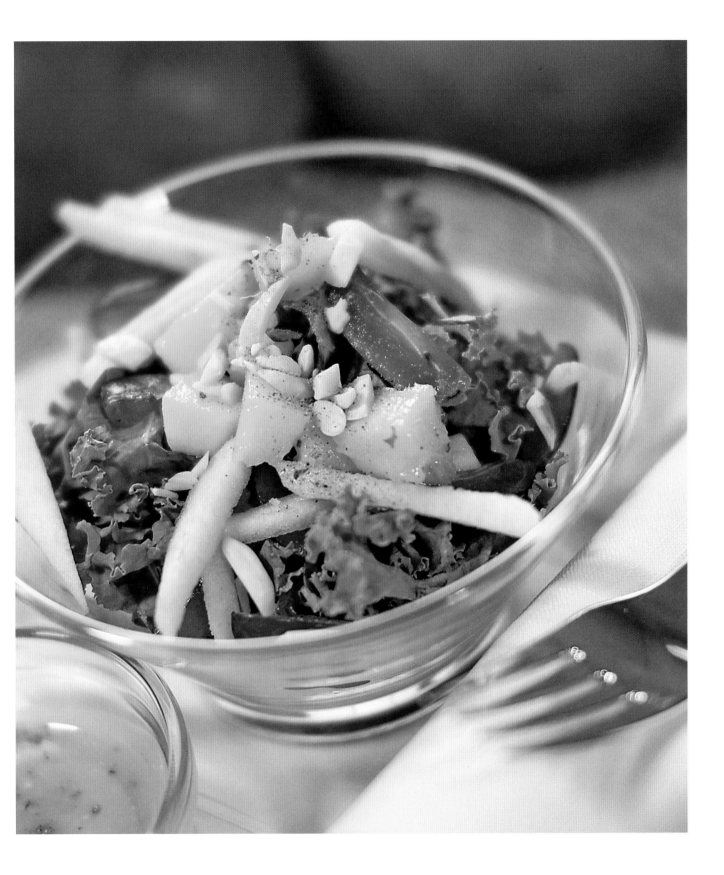

Blueberry Almond Salad

SERVES 2

1 banana

½ cup unsweetened soy, hemp, or almond milk

1 tablespoon raw almond butter

2 cups fresh or thawed frozen blueberries*

4 cups shredded romaine lettuce

* You can use strawberries, raspberries, or blackberries, too.

Blend banana, nondairy milk, and almond butter in a high-powered blender until smooth.

Toss shredded lettuce with the almond sauce and top with berries.

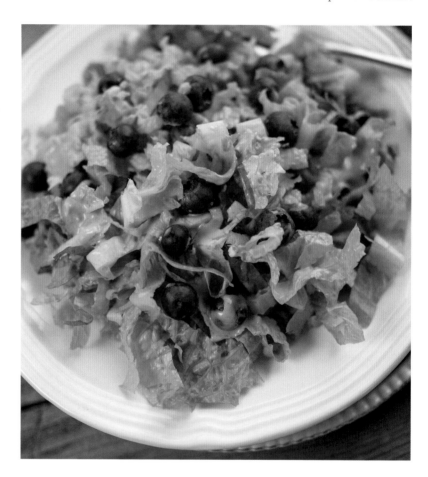

PER SERVING: CALORIES 235; PROTEIN 7g; CARBOHYDRATES 43g; TOTAL FAT 6.5g; SATURATED FAT 0.6g; SODIUM 41mg; FIBER 8.2g; BETA-CAROTENE 4,976mcg; VITAMIN C 23mg; CALCIUM 86mg; IRON 2.2mg; FOLATE 164mcg; MAGNESIUM 76mg; ZINC 0.9mg; SELENIUM 4.2mcg

Chopped Nutty Fruit and Vegetable Salad

No need for a salad dressing—the ingredients in this micro-chopped salad combine to provide a nicely balanced texture and flavor.

Place the apple, orange, and lemon in the bottom of a 14-cup food processor, and then add small pieces of lettuce, spinach, cabbage, broccoli, and carrots. Put the nuts on top. Chop coarsely with the S-shaped metal chopping blade.

SERVES 2

1 small tart apple, quartered

1 small orange, peeled and seeded

1 lemon, peeled and seeded

6 ounces romaine lettuce (about 3 cups chopped)

1 ounce spinach (about 1 cup chopped)

5 ounces green cabbage (about 2 cups chopped)

3 ounces broccoli (about 1 cup florets)

1 ounce carrots (about ½ carrot, chopped)

1 ounce walnuts

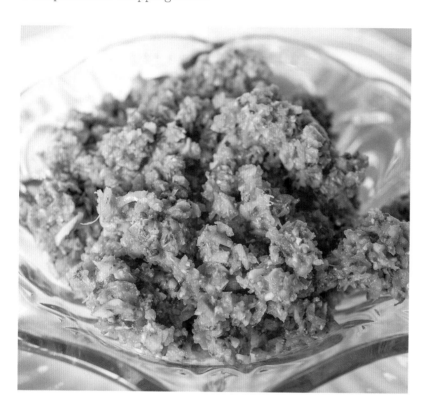

PER SERVING: CALORIES 238; PROTEIN 7g; CARBOHYDRATES 38g; TOTAL FAT 10.2g; SATURATED FAT 1g; SODIUM 57mg; FIBER 10.9g; BETA-CAROTENE 6,688mcg; VITAMIN C 133mg; CALCIUM 152mg; IRON 2.7mg; FOLATE 247mcg; MAGNESIUM 79mg; ZINC 1.2mg; SELENIUM 2.6mcg

DIPS, CHIPS, AND ACCOMPANIMENTS

To change things up, begin your meal with a healthful bean dip or salsa and a variety of colorful raw vegetables.

Starting your meal with veggies and dip is a fun alternative to having a salad. Dips make it easy to eat lots of raw vegetables, which will fill you up and prevent overeating. Tomatoes, zucchini, cucumber, carrot sticks, snow pea pods, raw string beans, raw broccoli, and raw cauliflower all taste great with a delicious dip.

Dips also make easy and delicious fillings for wraps or pitas when combined with shredded lettuce, chopped tomato, and sliced red onion and avocado.

You don't need to feel guilty about serving and enjoying Crispy Kale Chips or Italian Chickpea Popcorn. They are festive side dishes for kids of all ages. Pair them with a bean burger or a hearty bowl of soup, or sprinkle them on your salads.

Back-to-Basics Guacamole

2 ripe avocados, peeled and pitted

½ cup finely chopped onion

1 small tomato, chopped

1 clove garlic, diced

¼ cup minced fresh cilantro

2 tablespoons fresh lime juice

¼ teaspoon ground cumin

¼ teaspoon freshly ground black pepper

Using a fork, mash the avocados in a small bowl. Add the remaining ingredients and stir well.

PER SERVING: CALORIES 130; PROTEIN 2g; CARBOHYDRATES 10g; TOTAL FAT 10.6g; SATURATED FAT 1.5g; SODIUM 8mg; FIBER 5.4g; BETA-CAROTENE 188mcg; VITAMIN C 13mg; CALCIUM 21mg; IRON 0.7mg; FOLATE 69mcg; MAGNESIUM 26mg; ZINC 0.6mg; SELENIUM 0.5mcg

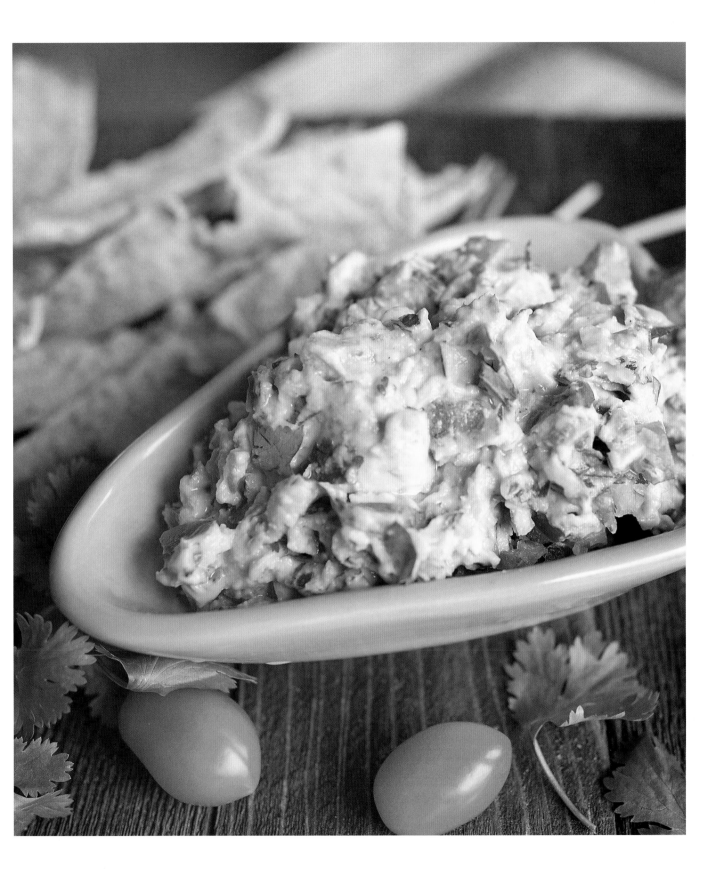

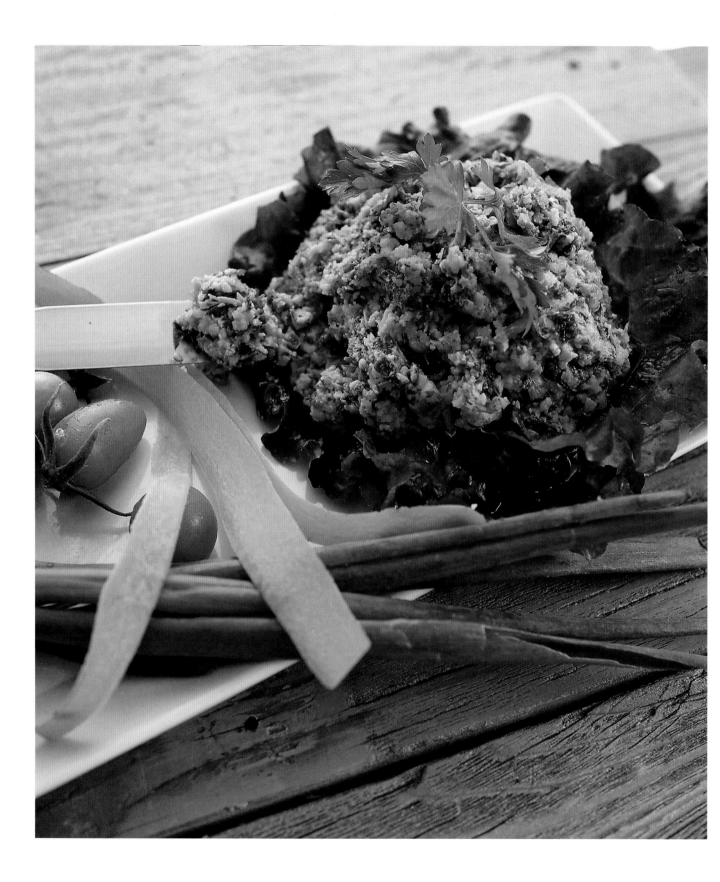

Perfect Pesto

Use this tasty pesto as a dip for raw veggies or as a topping for cooked vegetables or bean pasta. Store leftovers in the refrigerator; they will keep for several days.

In a food processor or blender, pulse walnuts and pine nuts until coarsely chopped. Add remaining ingredients and pulse until all ingredients are chopped and well combined.

SERVES 6

⅔ cup walnuts or raw almonds

⅔ cup pine nuts

1 cup fresh basil leaves, packed

⅔ cup fresh parsley, cilantro, or arugula leaves, packed

3 cloves garlic

1 teaspoon Bragg Liquid Aminos

2 tablespoons lemon juice

½ cup chopped tomato

PER SERVING: CALORIES 185; PROTEIN 5g; CARBOHYDRATES 6g; TOTAL FAT 15.8g; SATURATED FAT 1.2g; CHOLESTEROL 0.1mg; SODIUM 86mg; FIBER 2.5g; BETA-CAROTENE 629mcg; VITAMIN C 15mg; CALCIUM 53mg; IRON 2mg; FOLATE 26mcg; MAGNESIUM 78mg; ZINC 1.5mg; SELENIUM 0.6mcg

Red Bean Salsa with Baked Pita Chips

SERVES 6 (4 CUPS)

1 ½ cups cooked or 1 (15-ounce) can low-sodium or no-salt-added kidney beans, drained

4 plum tomatoes, chopped

¼ cup chopped red onion

½ red or green bell pepper, chopped

¼ cup no-salt-added tomato paste*

¼ cup raw almond butter

2 tablespoons balsamic vinegar

½ teaspoon chili powder, or to taste

½ teaspoon dried oregano

6 (100% whole grain) pitas

....

Look for tomato paste packaged in non-BPA-containing glass jars.

Place all ingredients except pitas in a bowl and mix together with a fork.

To make baked pita chips, preheat oven to 300°F. Separate the layers of the pita pockets and cut into triangles. Arrange on a baking sheet and bake 10 minutes or until slightly crisp.

Serve with baked pita chips and raw veggies.

PER SERVING: CALORIES 148; PROTEIN 7g; CARBOHYDRATES 18g; TOTAL FAT 6.2g; SATURATED FAT 0.5g; SODIUM 16mg; FIBER 5.8g; BETA-CAROTENE 480mcg; VITAMIN C 22mg; CALCIUM 63mg; IRON 2.3mg; FOLATE 77mcg; MAGNESIUM 61mg; ZINC 1mg; SELENIUM 1.5mcg

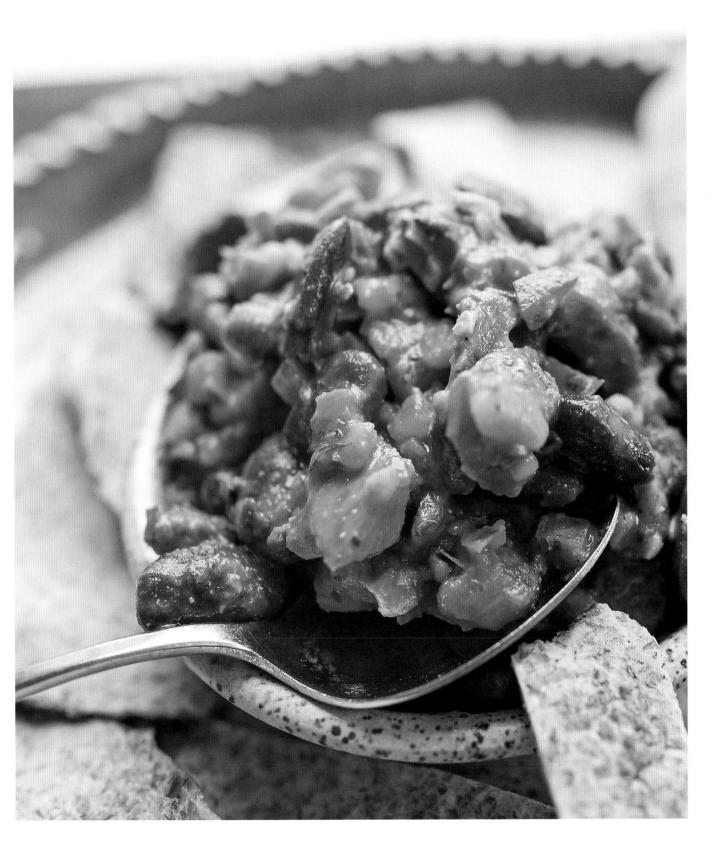

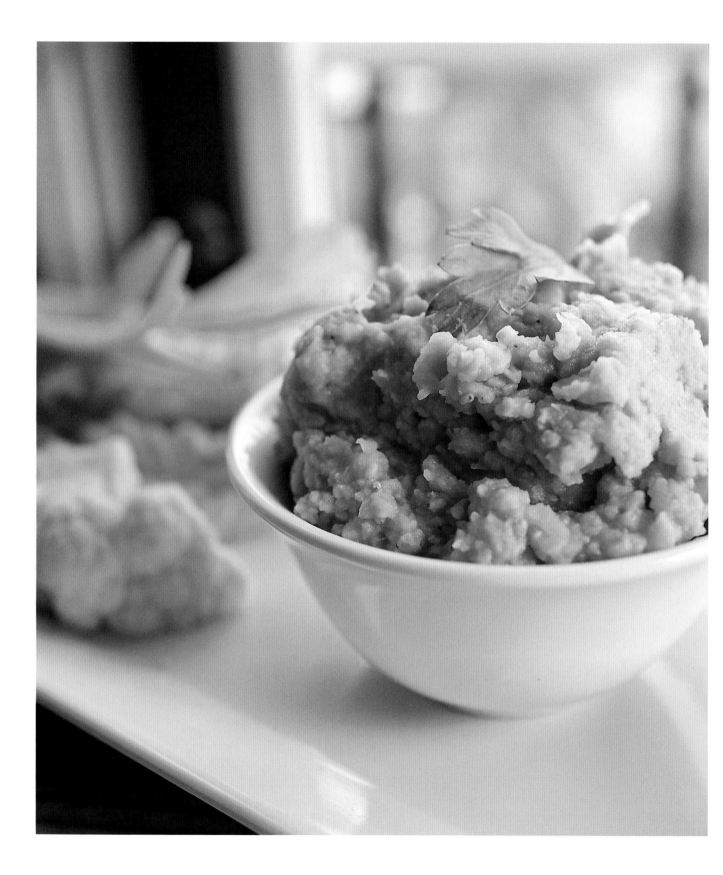

Super Simple Hummus

Blend all ingredients in a high-powered blender or food processor. Add 1–2 tablespoons water if needed to adjust consistency.

Can be refrigerated in an airtight container for up to 4 days.

SERVES 4

1 ½ cups cooked or 1 (15-ounce) can no-salt-added or low-sodium chickpeas, drained

2 tablespoons lemon juice

3 tablespoons unhulled sesame seeds

1 clove garlic, minced

½ teaspoon ground cumin

PER SERVING: CALORIES 130; PROTEIN 6g; CARBOHYDRATES 19g; TOTAL FAT 3.9g; SATURATED FAT 0.5g; SODIUM 5mg; FIBER 5.3g; BETA-CAROTENE 12mcg; VITAMIN C 4mg; CALCIUM 78mg; IRON 2.6mg; FOLATE 112mcg; MAGNESIUM 47mg; ZINC 1.3mg; SELENIUM 4mcg

Nutri-tella

1 cup raw hazelnuts

2–3 medjool dates or 4–6 regular dates, pitted

2 ½ tablespoons natural cocoa powder

1 tablespoon ground chia seeds

1 teaspoon alcohol-free vanilla extract

½ cup coconut water or more as needed to facilitate blending

No need to feel guilty about indulging in this delicious chocolate hazelnut spread. Spread it on apples, bananas, or romaine lettuce leaves.

Pulse the hazelnuts in a food processor until the consistency of hazelnut meal.

Transfer the processed nuts to a high-powered blender and add the dates, cocoa powder, ground chia seeds, vanilla, and just enough coconut water so that the mixture moves. Blend at high speed until smooth and fluffy.

Refrigerate for several hours to thicken.

PER SERVING: CALORIES 134; PROTEIN 3g; CARBOHYDRATES 9g; TOTAL FAT 10.7g; SATURATED FAT 0.9g; SODIUM 16mg; FIBER 3g; BETA-CAROTENE 7mcg; VITAMIN C 1mg; CALCIUM 33mg; IRON 1.2mg; FOLATE 21mcg; MAGNESIUM 45mg; ZINC 0.6mg; SELENIUM 1.1mcg

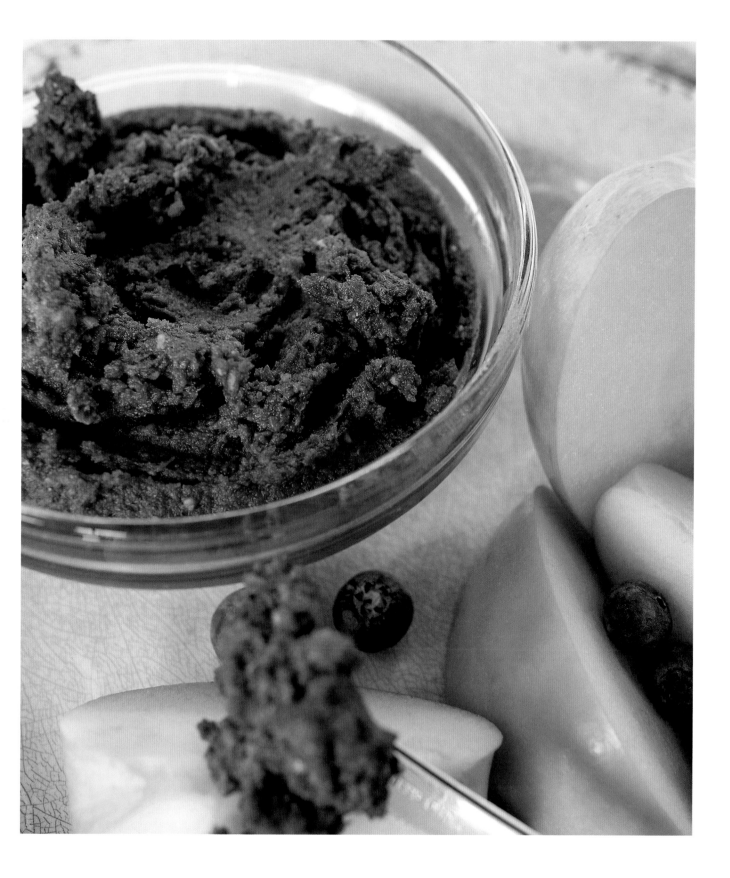

Quick Baba Ganoush

SERVES 4

1 (1 ½-pound) eggplant

2 cloves garlic, chopped

2 tablespoons fresh lemon juice

1 tablespoon tahini or unhulled sesame seeds

1 tablespoon chopped flat leaf parsley

Baba ganoush is a Middle Eastern spread and dip that is similar to hummus, but it is made with eggplant instead of chickpeas. Serve it with raw vegetables or spread it on a veggie wrap.

Preheat oven to 400°F. Prick eggplant with a fork and place on a cookie sheet. Bake 50 minutes, or until soft, turning occasionally.

Let eggplant cool to touch. Peel. Put all ingredients in the food processor and puree until smooth. Chill before serving.

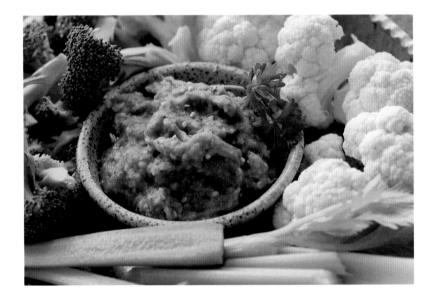

PER SERVING: CALORIES 66; PROTEIN 3g; CARBOHYDRATES 12g; TOTAL FAT 2.2g; SATURATED FAT 0.3g; SODIUM 7mg; FIBER 6.2g; BETA-CAROTENE 75mcg; VITAMIN C 8mg; CALCIUM 36mg; IRON 0.6mg; FOLATE 44mcg; MAGNESIUM 29mg; ZINC 0.5mg; SELENIUM 0.7mcg

Crispy Kale Chips

Preheat oven to 225°F or lowest setting available.

Tear kale into uniform, chip-size pieces.

Mix a dressing by blending raw cashews or almonds with water or nondairy milk and your choice of (or a combination of) flavor options. Adjust seasoning amounts to your taste.

Using sparingly, hand massage dressing into the kale. Then spread kale evenly on a nonstick baking sheet.

Bake 50 minutes or until crispy and dry, tossing occasionally to prevent burning.

If using a lower temperature, or a dehydrator, cooking for a longer time is necessary: 8–10 hours for a temperature of 125°F.

SERVES 6

3 bunches kale, tough stems and center ribs removed

½ cup raw cashews or almonds

⅓ cup water or soy, hemp, or almond milk.

Creative flavor options

1 tablespoon balsamic vinegar, apple cider vinegar, or lemon juice

2 tablespoons unfortified nutritional yeast

1 teaspoon garlic powder

1 teaspoon onion powder

1 teaspoon VegiZest or MatoZest, Mrs. Dash seasoning blend, or other no-salt seasoning blend

1 teaspoon chili powder

¼ teaspoon black pepper

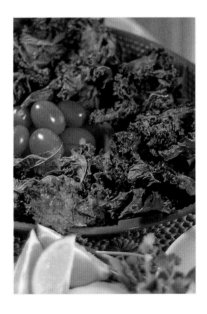

TIP: The human body was designed to get its optimal level of sodium from a natural diet of unsalted foods. Most Americans consume about six times more sodium than they need. The high blood pressure that results from a lifetime of salt exposure is a major cause of the 1.5 million heart attacks each year.

PER SERVING: CALORIES 115; PROTEIN 6g; CARBOHYDRATES 10g; TOTAL FAT 6.6g; SATURATED FAT 0.6g; SODIUM 40mg; FIBER 3.2g; BETA-CAROTENE 4,495mcg; VITAMIN C 59mg; CALCIUM 114mg; IRON 1.6mg; FOLATE 25mcg; MAGNESIUM 55mg; ZINC 1.2mg; SELENIUM 1mcg

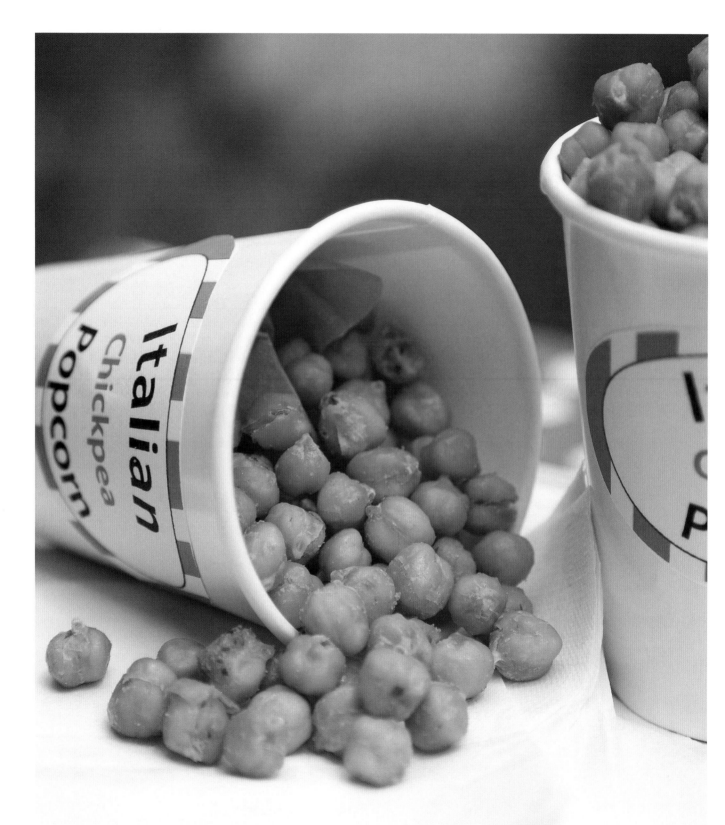

Italian Chickpea Popcorn

These crunchy chickpeas are great by themselves, or you can also use them to top soups or salads.

Preheat oven to 350°F.

Mix chickpeas with remaining ingredients.

Spread on a baking sheet and bake 40–45 minutes or until crispy, stirring occasionally.

SERVES 6

1 ½ cups cooked or 1 (15-ounce) can no-salt-added or low-sodium chickpeas, drained and rinsed

1 teaspoon ground cumin

1 teaspoon garlic powder

1 teaspoon oregano

Pinch of cayenne pepper, or to taste

1 teaspoon olive oil

PER SERVING: CALORIES 67; PROTEIN 4g; CARBOHYDRATES 11g; TOTAL FAT 1.1g; SATURATED FAT 0.1g; SODIUM 3mg; FIBER 3.1g; BETA-CAROTENE 7mcg; VITAMIN C 1mg; CALCIUM 20mg; IRON 1.2mg; FOLATE 71mcg; MAGNESIUM 20mg; ZINC 0.6mg; SELENIUM 1.5mcg

SOUPS AND STEWS

*When made with healthful ingredients,
soup is the ideal one-pot meal.*

Soups are an important part of my Nutritarian diet. It is easy to combine a variety of green leafy vegetables, mushrooms, onions, beans, and other healthy ingredients all in one pot. When vegetables are simmered together in a soup, all the nutrients are retained in the liquid, and the gentle heat prevents nutrient loss.

Get in the habit of making a pot of soup once or twice a week. There is a soup for every taste and preference. Don't be afraid to switch around vegetables or substitute different types of beans. Adjust spices and herbs to your taste or add additional seasonings if you like.

I often blend nuts into my soups to provide a rich flavor and creamy texture. You can choose to blend the entire soup, or just a portion if you prefer a chunky texture. People with nut allergies can just blend the soup without adding any nuts.

Soups also make great leftovers for lunch, or for those nights when you are too busy to cook.

Buenas Noches Black Bean Soup

1 large onion, chopped

2 cups chopped celery

2 cups chopped carrots

4 cloves garlic, chopped

1 tablespoon ground cumin

2 teaspoons chili powder

¼ teaspoon black pepper

6 cups water

1 tablespoon VegiZest or other no-salt seasoning, adjusted to taste

6 cups cooked or 4 (15-ounce) cans low-sodium or no-salt-added black beans, divided

1 (16-ounce) jar mild picante sauce or salsa, no-salt-added or low-sodium*

2 cups thawed frozen corn

1 ½ cups diced tomatoes

....

* salt-free Tex-Mex Salsa is available at www.drfuhrman.com/shop.

In a large soup pot, combine onion, celery, carrots, garlic, cumin, chili powder, black pepper, water, VegiZest, and 3 cups beans. Bring to a boil, reduce heat, and simmer for 15 minutes.

Place remaining 3 cups beans and the picante sauce or salsa in a blender or food processor. Blend on high speed until smooth. Stir into soup mixture along with corn and tomatoes.

Simmer for an additional 15 minutes.

PER SERVING: CALORIES 354; PROTEIN 20g; CARBOHYDRATES 69g; TOTAL FAT 2.5g; SATURATED FAT 0.5g; SODIUM 127mg; FIBER 21.4g; BETA-CAROTENE 4,576mcg; VITAMIN C 28mg; CALCIUM 134mg; IRON 5.9mg; FOLATE 330mcg; MAGNESIUM 171mg; ZINC 2.8mg; SELENIUM 3.8mcg

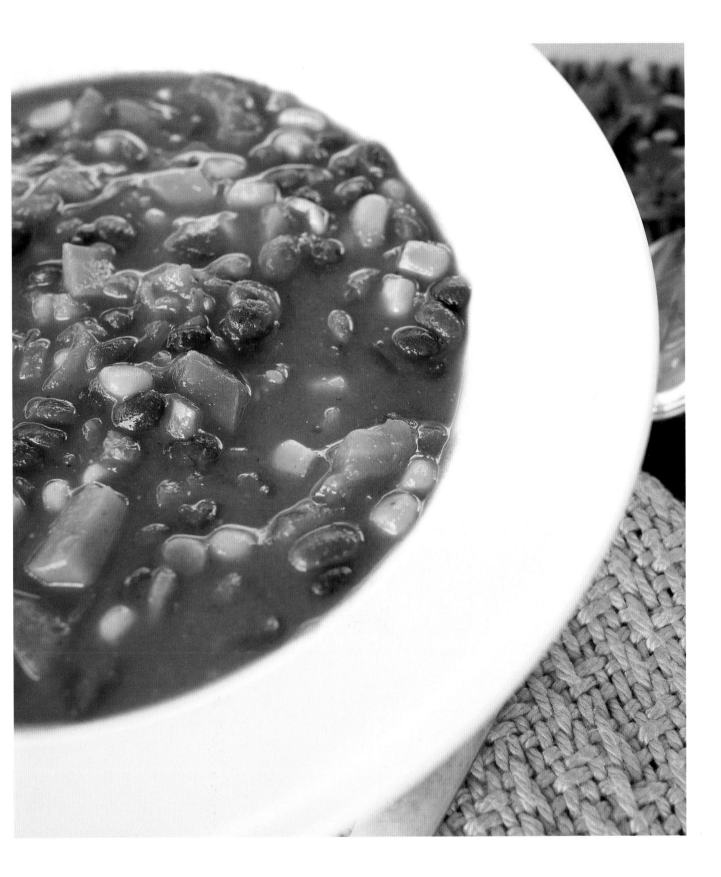

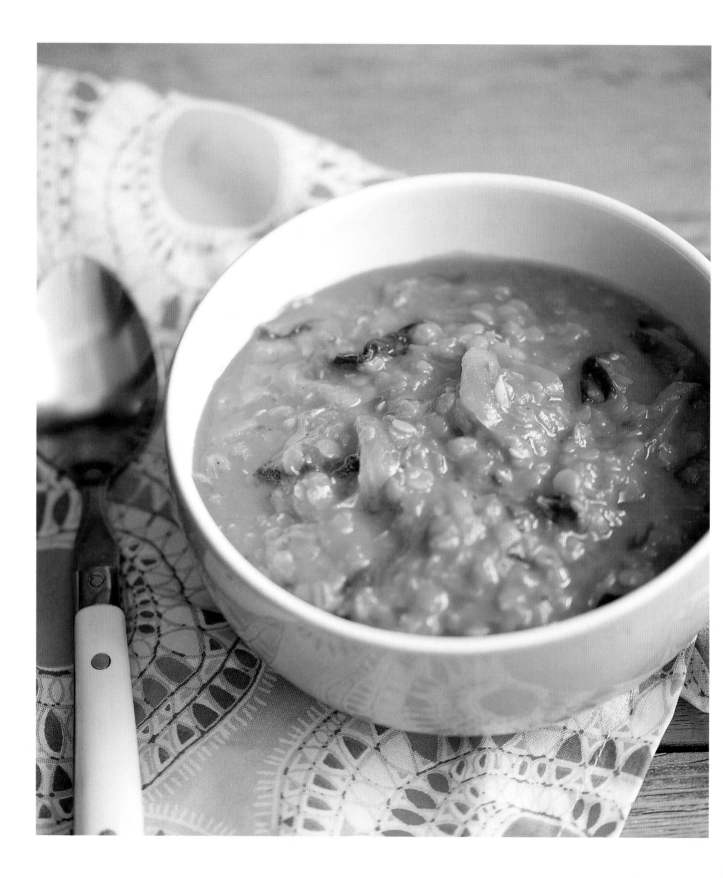

Carrot and Red Lentil Soup

Heat 2–3 tablespoons water in a soup pot and water-sauté onions and garlic until tender. Add carrot juice, vegetable broth, and lentils. Bring to a boil, lower heat, and simmer, covered, until the lentils are soft, about 50–60 minutes.

Stir in baby kale or spinach and heat until wilted.

Add lemon juice and chopped parsley.

SERVES 6

3–4 large sweet onions, chopped

2 cloves garlic, chopped

4 cups carrot juice

4 cups low-sodium or no-salt-added vegetable broth

1 pound red lentils

5 ounces baby kale or spinach

2 tablespoons fresh lemon juice, or to taste

¼ cup chopped parsley

PER SERVING: CALORIES 394; PROTEIN 23g; CARBOHYDRATES 74g; TOTAL FAT 1.3g; SATURATED FAT 0.2g; SODIUM 215mg; FIBER 26.6g; BETA-CAROTENE 16,961mcg; VITAMIN C 58mg; CALCIUM 156mg; IRON 7.5mg; FOLATE 399mcg; MAGNESIUM 134mg; ZINC 4.2mg; SELENIUM 8.1mcg

"Cream" of Broccoli Soup

SERVES 6

1 onion, chopped

2 cloves garlic, chopped

5 cups low-sodium or no-salt-added vegetable broth or carrot juice

4 turnips, peeled and chopped

1 bunch kale, tough stems removed, chopped

4 bunches broccoli, coarsely chopped

1 cup water

½ cup raw cashews

Turnips, an often-overlooked cruciferous vegetable, provide a hearty consistency and slightly peppery flavor.

Heat 2–3 tablespoons water in a soup pot and water-sauté onion and garlic until softened.

Add vegetable broth or carrot juice, turnips, kale, broccoli, and water. Bring to a boil, reduce heat, and simmer until turnips and vegetables are tender, about 20–25 minutes.

Blend half the soup with the cashews, return mixture to pot, and reheat.

TIP: Eating large volumes of healthy food is what makes the Nutritarian program so effective for losing weight and preventing and reversing disease. By eating so much of the "good stuff," you will naturally desire less low-nutrient food. As a consequence of eating a high-nutrient diet and getting fueled with antioxidants and phytochemicals, you gradually and naturally optimize your health and lose your desire to overeat.

PER SERVING: CALORIES 339; PROTEIN 19g; CARBOHYDRATES 61g; TOTAL FAT 7.2g; SATURATED FAT 1.2g; SODIUM 348mg; FIBER 16g; BETA-CAROTENE 22,113mcg; VITAMIN C 468mg; CALCIUM 328mg; IRON 5.7mg; FOLATE 319mcg; MAGNESIUM 175mg; ZINC 3.2mg; SELENIUM 15.8mcg

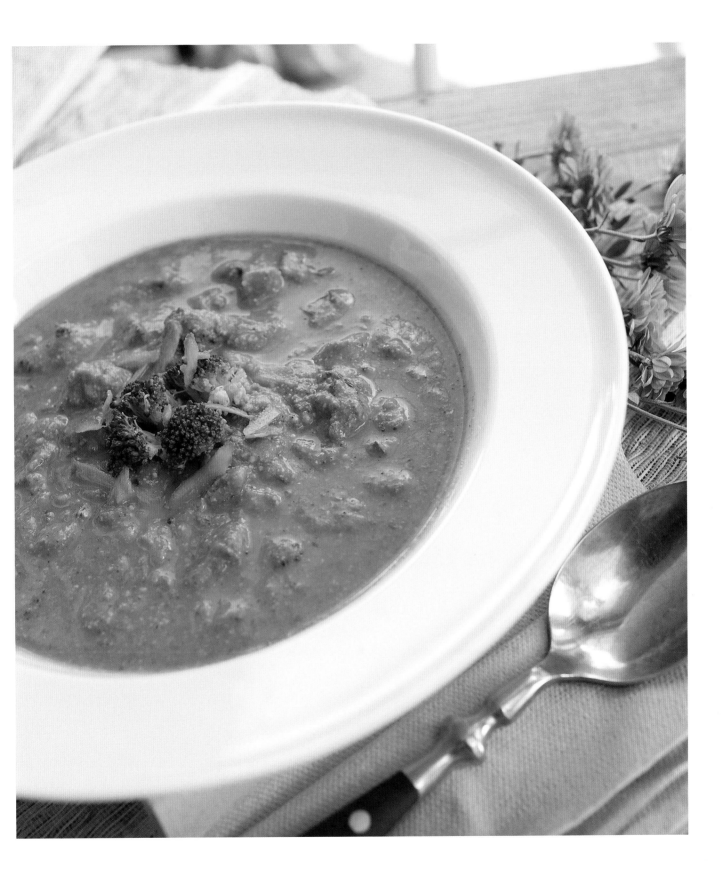

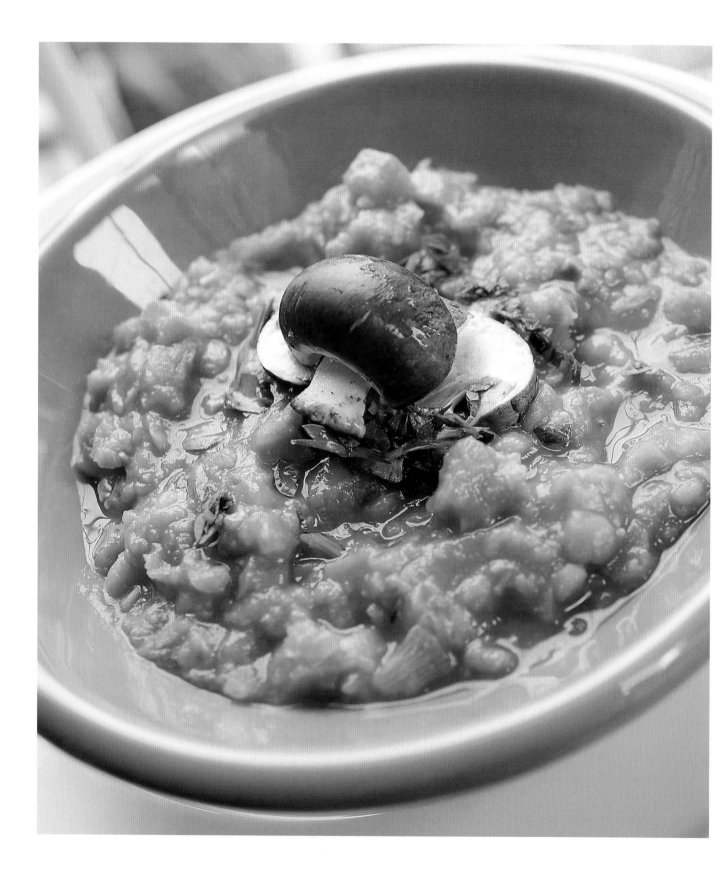

Easy Split Pea Stew

In a large soup pot, combine split peas, broth, bay leaf, thyme, and cumin. Bring to boiling, reduce heat, and simmer, covered, for 45 minutes, stirring occasionally.

Stir in onion, celery, carrots, mushrooms, and garlic. Return to boiling, reduce heat, and simmer, covered, for 20–25 minutes more, or until vegetables are tender.

Stir in baby spinach and cook until wilted.

Discard bay leaf.

Stir in sherry.

SERVES 6

1 pound dry split peas, rinsed

8 cups low-sodium or no-salt-added vegetable broth

1 bay leaf

½ teaspoon dried thyme

1 teaspoon dried cumin

1 medium onion, chopped

4 stalks celery, thinly sliced

3 medium carrots, chopped

1 cup chopped mushrooms

2 cloves garlic, minced

4 cups packed baby spinach

2 tablespoons dry sherry or sherry vinegar

TIP: Onions and mushrooms add great flavor to all kinds of dishes and also have well-documented anticancer and immunity-building properties.

PER SERVING: CALORIES 286; PROTEIN 20g; CARBOHYDRATES 52g; TOTAL FAT 1.1g; SATURATED FAT 0.2g; SODIUM 53mg; FIBER 20.8g; BETA-CAROTENE 3,743mcg; VITAMIN C 5mg; CALCIUM 79mg; IRON 4mg; FOLATE 222mcg; MAGNESIUM 100mg; ZINC 2.6mg; SELENIUM 4.6mcg

Gingery Red Lentil Butternut Soup

SERVES 6

4 cups no-salt-added or low-sodium vegetable stock

12 ounces butternut squash, chopped

10 ounces frozen, chopped spinach

1 ½ cups no-salt-added packaged diced tomatoes (or 4 fresh tomatoes, diced)

¾ cup dried red lentils

2 teaspoons grated ginger, or more to taste

1 tablespoon minced dried onion

1 teaspoon ground cumin

1 teaspoon no-salt seasoning blend, adjusted to taste

1 ½ cups cooked or 1 (15-ounce) can no-salt-added or low-sodium white beans, drained

Precut butternut squash is a great time saver. It is available in many food markets.

Put all ingredients except white beans in a slow cooker or a pot on the stove top. Simmer until lentils are tender, about 7 hours in slow cooker on low or 1 hour on stove.

Add white beans and cook an additional 10 minutes.

If you want this to be more soupy, decrease the red lentils to ½ cup.

> PER SERVING: CALORIES 161; PROTEIN 11g; CARBOHYDRATES 31g; TOTAL FAT 1.1g; SATURATED FAT 0.1g; SODIUM 87mg; FIBER 11.2g; BETA-CAROTENE 6,099mcg; VITAMIN C 31mg; CALCIUM 138mg; IRON 4.2mg; FOLATE 233mcg; MAGNESIUM 111mg; ZINC 1.8mg; SELENIUM 5.7mcg

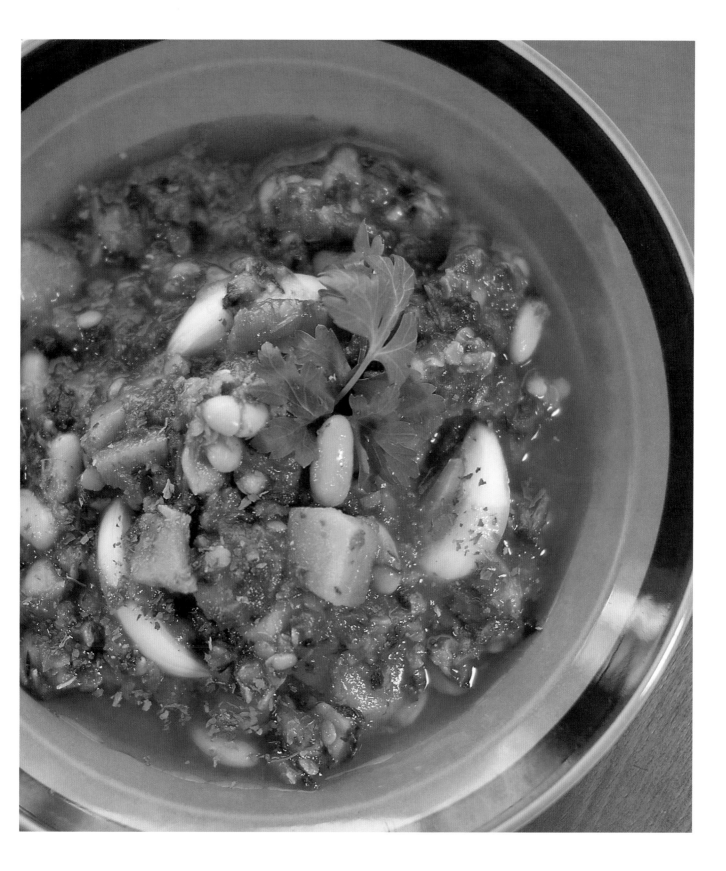

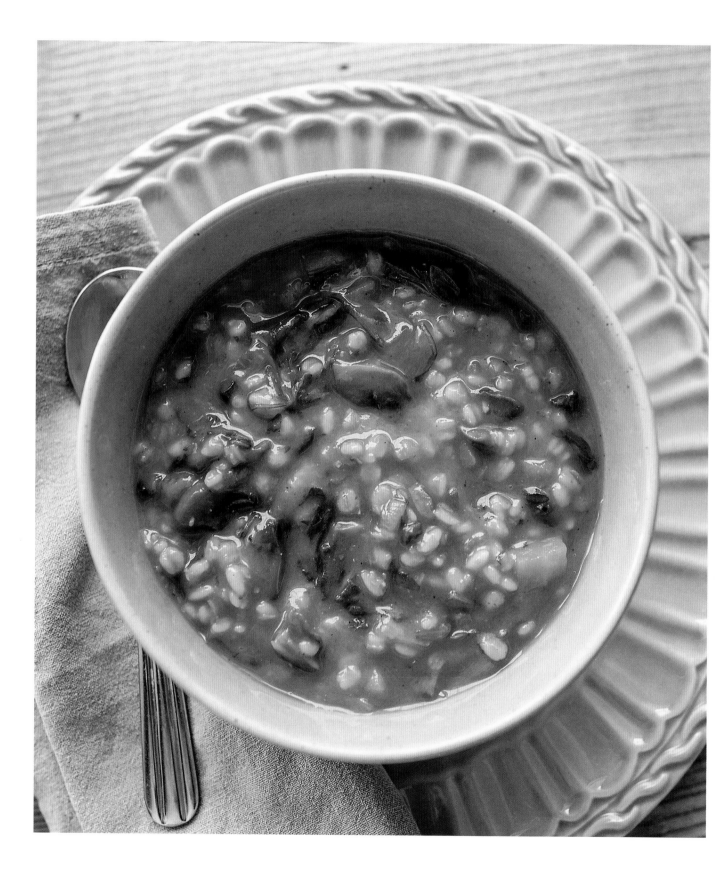

Mushroom and Barley Soup

The classic combination of barley and mushrooms makes a satisfying and soothing soup.

Heat ¼ cup water in a large soup pot and water-sauté onions, carrots, celery, and garlic until softened, about 6 minutes. Add mushrooms and Bragg Liquid Aminos and cook until mushrooms release their juices, about 5 minutes.

Add barley, vegetable broth, black pepper, and thyme, bring to a boil, reduce heat, cover, and simmer for 60 minutes or until barley is tender.

Stir in arugula and heat until wilted.

SERVES 4

1 medium onion, chopped

1 cup chopped carrots

½ cup chopped celery

3 cloves garlic, minced

20 ounces mushrooms, sliced

1 teaspoon Bragg Liquid Aminos

1 cup whole grain barley*

8 cups low-sodium or no-salt-added vegetable broth

¼ teaspoon ground black pepper, or to taste

½ teaspoon dried thyme

2 cups arugula

* *Hulled barley and hull-less barley are two different varieties of barley; both are considered whole grains. Quicker-cooking pearl barley has been refined and is not a whole grain.*

PER SERVING: CALORIES 255; PROTEIN 11g; CARBOHYDRATES 51g; TOTAL FAT 1.8g; SATURATED FAT 0.3g; SODIUM 379mg; FIBER 11.3g; BETA-CAROTENE 2,844mcg; VITAMIN C 10mg; CALCIUM 113mg; IRON 3.8mg; FOLATE 60mcg; MAGNESIUM 88mg; ZINC 2.2mg; SELENIUM 27.1mcg

Cauliflower and Sweet Potato Soup

SERVES 4

2 cups chopped onions

2 medium sweet potatoes, peeled and diced

1 tablespoon ground cumin

1 teaspoon ground coriander

1 teaspoon ground fennel

¼ teaspoon cayenne pepper, or to taste

1 medium head cauliflower, chopped

6 cups no-salt-added or low-sodium vegetable broth

2 tablespoons fresh lemon juice

1 large tomato, chopped

In a large soup pot, water-sauté onions until tender. Add sweet potatoes, cumin, coriander, fennel, and cayenne pepper and cook for 1 minute.

Add cauliflower and vegetable broth, bring to a boil, reduce heat, cover, and simmer for 20 minutes or until vegetables are tender.

Working in batches, add soup to a high-powered blender and puree until smooth.

Return to pot, add lemon juice, and reheat. Add additional vegetable broth or water if needed to adjust consistency.

Garnish with chopped tomato.

PER SERVING: CALORIES 156; PROTEIN 5g; CARBOHYDRATES 33g; TOTAL FAT 1.1g; SATURATED FAT 0.2g; SODIUM 292mg; FIBER 7g; BETA-CAROTENE 5,772mcg; VITAMIN C 86mg; CALCIUM 129mg; IRON 3.1mg; FOLATE 110mcg; MAGNESIUM 59mg; ZINC 0.9mg; SELENIUM 1.8mcg

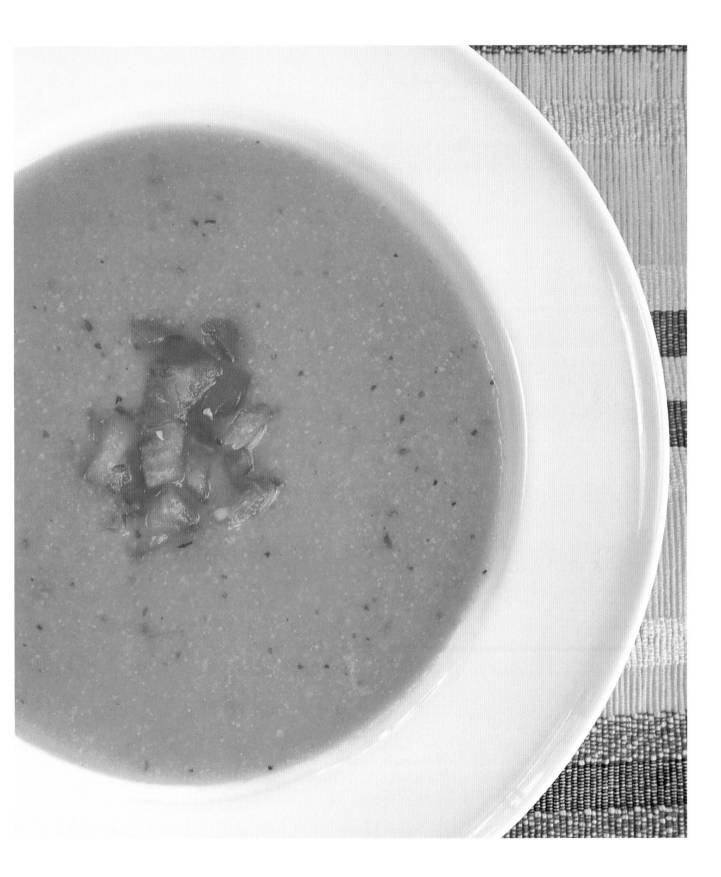

Eggplant and Black Bean Stew

SERVES 6

2 cups dried black beans, soaked overnight

1 ½ cups low-sodium vegetable broth

1 ½ cups water

1 teaspoon cumin

1 ½ teaspoons oregano

3 cloves garlic, crushed

1 small eggplant, peeled and cubed (about 2 ¼ cups)

4 stalks celery, chopped

2 cups finely chopped tomatoes

⅓ cup tomato paste*

....

Look for tomato paste packaged in non-BPA-containing glass jars.

Use a pressure cooker to quickly and easily cook dry beans.

Combine black beans, vegetable broth, water, cumin, oregano, and crushed garlic in pressure cooker. With lid off, start to heat as you prepare the eggplant and celery.

Add the celery and then the eggplant on top. Eggplant will not be fully submerged and will stick up above the liquid. Lock lid into place, and bring to full pressure on high heat. Maintain pressure for 12 minutes, and then allow pressure to release naturally.

When pressure has released, stir in the diced tomatoes and tomato paste.

PER SERVING: CALORIES 274; PROTEIN 16g; CARBOHYDRATES 52g; TOTAL FAT 1.4g; SATURATED FAT 0.3g; SODIUM 75mg; FIBER 14.6g; BETA-CAROTENE 492mcg; VITAMIN C 14mg; CALCIUM 129mg; IRON 4.6mg; FOLATE 325mcg; MAGNESIUM 140mg; ZINC 2.8mg; SELENIUM 3.4mcg

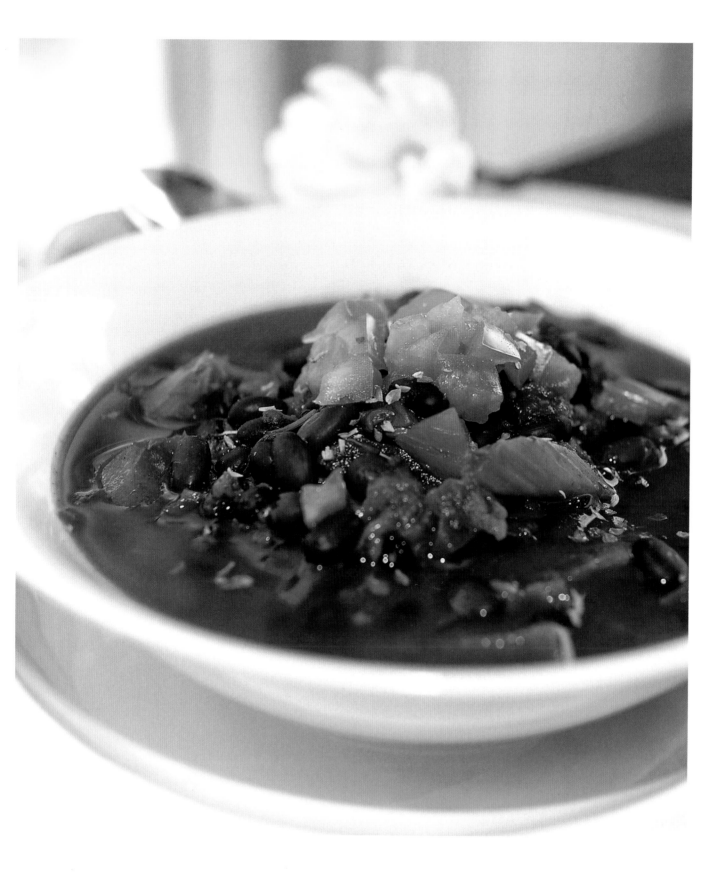

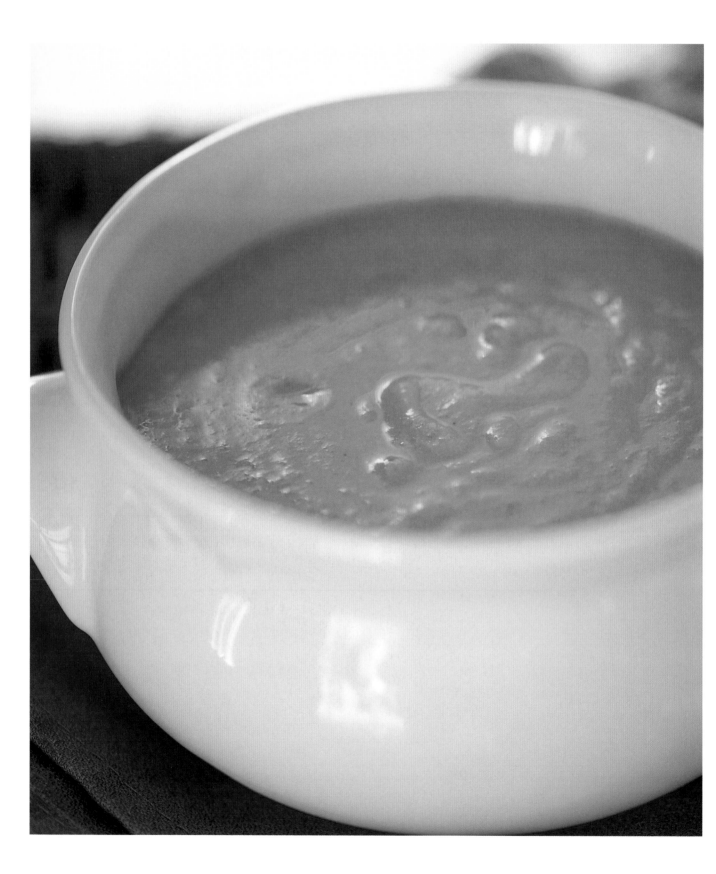

Creamy Cauliflower Soup

Heat 2–3 tablespoons water in a soup pot and water-sauté onion and garlic until soft. Add cauliflower, carrot juice, and 4 cups vegetable broth; bring to a boil, reduce heat, and simmer for 25 minutes or until cauliflower is very tender.

Working in batches, blend soup with cashews in a high-powered blender.

Return to soup pot and reheat before serving.

Season with no-salt seasoning, curry powder, and turmeric. Stir in dill. If desired, add additional vegetable broth to adjust consistency.

SERVES 4

1 medium onion, chopped

2 cloves garlic

1 head cauliflower, chopped

2 cups carrot juice

4–5 cups low-sodium or no-salt-added vegetable broth

½ cup raw cashews

1 teaspoon no-salt seasoning blend, adjusted to taste

¼ teaspoon curry powder

¼ teaspoon ground turmeric

¼ cup chopped fresh dill

TIP: Cruciferous vegetables are not only the most powerful anti-cancer foods in existence, but also the most micronutrient-dense of all vegetables. The cruciferous vegetables include arugula, kale, collards, bok choy, broccoli, cauliflower, cabbage, Brussels sprouts, mustard greens, and watercress.

PER SERVING: CALORIES 209; PROTEIN 8g; CARBOHYDRATES 29g; TOTAL FAT 8.1g; SATURATED FAT 1.5g; SODIUM 263mg; FIBER 5.1g; BETA-CAROTENE 10,979mcg; VITAMIN C 84mg; CALCIUM 104mg; IRON 3mg; FOLATE 102mcg; MAGNESIUM 94mg; ZINC 1.7mg; SELENIUM 5.4mcg

Quick and Easy Kale and White Bean Stew

SERVES 6

2 bunches kale, tough stems removed and leaves coarsely chopped

¼ cup water

1 medium onion, chopped

2 cloves garlic, minced

No-salt seasoning blend, adjusted to taste, or 1 tablespoon MatoZest

¼ teaspoon ground black pepper

¼ teaspoon crushed red pepper, or to taste

3 cups cooked or 2 (15-ounce) cans low-sodium or no-salt-added cannellini or other white beans, drained

3 cups diced tomatoes

2 cups vegetable broth, low-sodium or no-salt-added, or more if needed to achieve desired consistency

Add kale and water to a soup pot, cover and cook over medium heat for 10 minutes or until kale is tender, stirring occasionally.

Add onion, garlic, seasoning blend, black pepper, and red pepper. Continue to cook, uncovered, for 5–7 more minutes.

Add beans, tomatoes, and vegetable broth and bring to boil. Reduce heat and simmer covered for 15–20 minutes, stirring occasionally.

PER SERVING: CALORIES 178; PROTEIN 12g; CARBOHYDRATES 34g; TOTAL FAT 0.9g; SATURATED FAT 0.2g; SODIUM 37mg; FIBER 8.7g; BETA-CAROTENE 4,780mcg; VITAMIN C 72mg; CALCIUM 167mg; IRON 4.6mg; FOLATE 108mcg; MAGNESIUM 88mg; ZINC 1.7mg; SELENIUM 1.9mcg

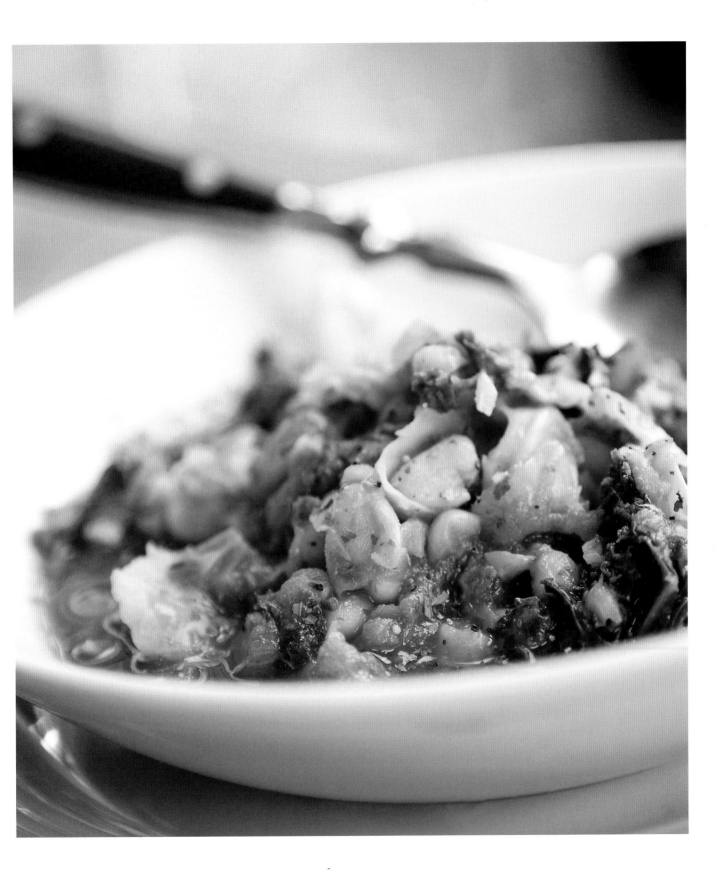

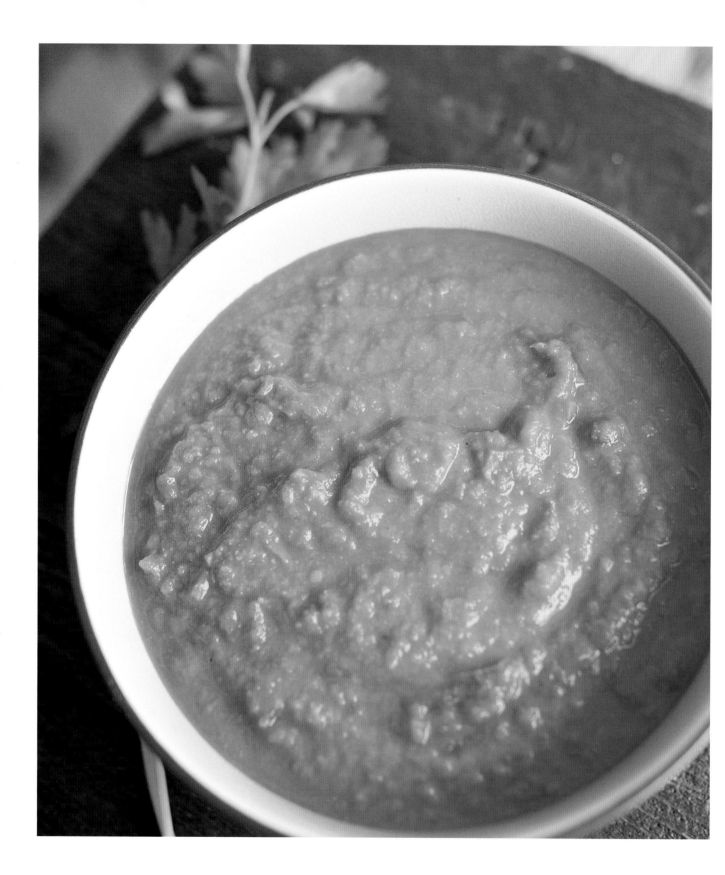

Quick and Spicy Tomato Bisque

Water-sauté onion over medium heat until softened. Add garlic and red pepper flakes, cooking and stirring until fragrant. Add tomatoes, seasoning blend, carrot juice, and sun-dried tomatoes. Bring to a low boil and simmer over low heat for 10 minutes.

Remove from heat and carefully pour into a high-powered blender. Blend on low speed, letting steam escape as necessary. Gradually increase speed to medium and add cashews. Blend until combined.

Return to stove, bring back to low simmer, then serve.

Serve by itself or over steamed greens or mixed vegetables.

SERVES 2

½ cup diced onion

4 cloves garlic, minced

1 teaspoon red pepper flakes, or to taste

28 ounces no-salt-added packaged chopped tomatoes*

No-salt seasoning blend, adjusted to taste, or 2 tablespoons MatoZest

1 cup carrot juice

3 unsulfured, no-salt-added sun-dried tomatoes

⅓ cup raw cashews

....

Choose tomatoes packaged in BPA-free cartons.

PER SERVING: CALORIES 313; PROTEIN 12g; CARBOHYDRATES 44g; TOTAL FAT 13g; SATURATED FAT 2.5g; SODIUM 144mg; FIBER 6.1g; BETA-CAROTENE 12,154mcg; VITAMIN C 111mg; CALCIUM 132mg; IRON 5.8mg; FOLATE 109mcg; MAGNESIUM 139mg; ZINC 2.3mg; SELENIUM 7mcg

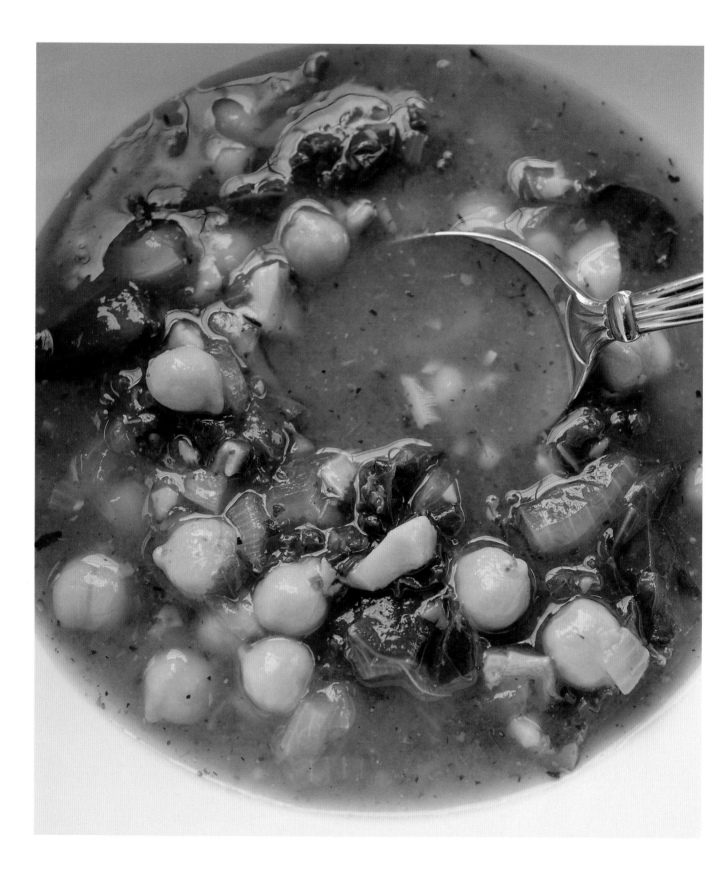

Ready-in-a-Flash Mushroom Soup

Water-sauté mushrooms and onions until dry and beginning to brown. Add spinach or kale and heat until wilted, adding more water if needed.

Puree white beans in a food processor or blender. Pour pureed beans over the mushroom mixture and season with MatoZest and pepper.

Add low-sodium vegetable broth to adjust consistency.

1 cup chopped mushrooms

½ onion, chopped

2 cups baby kale or spinach

1 ½ cups cooked or 1 (15-ounce) can low-sodium or no-salt-added white beans, drained

No-salt seasoning blend, adjusted to taste, or 1 tablespoon MatoZest

¼ teaspoon freshly ground black pepper, to taste

Low-sodium or no-salt-added vegetable broth as needed

PER SERVING: CALORIES 186; PROTEIN 11g; CARBOHYDRATES 36g; TOTAL FAT 0.9g; SATURATED FAT 0.2g; SODIUM 20mg; FIBER 9g; BETA-CAROTENE 192mcg; VITAMIN C 23mg; CALCIUM 90mg; IRON 4.2mg; FOLATE 65mcg; MAGNESIUM 88mg; ZINC 2mg; SELENIUM 14mcg

Spicy Corn and Red Pepper Soup

SERVES 8

8 ears sweet corn, kernels removed (or 4 cups frozen)

4 red bell peppers, diced

1 large onion, finely chopped

2 small red chili peppers, or to taste

2 tablespoons finely chopped cilantro

2 tablespoons arrowroot powder (or cornstarch)

4 cups low-sodium or no-salt-added vegetable broth

4 cups water

1 cup raw cashews

1 cup soy, hemp, or almond milk

Black pepper to taste

Savor the flavors of sweet corn and tomatoes in this creamy soup. If you don't like it spicy, cut back on the chili peppers.

Heat ¼ cup water in a soup pot over medium heat and add the corn kernels, red bell peppers, onion, and chili peppers and stir well. Reduce heat and cook, covered, for 10 minutes or until peppers start to soften, stirring occasionally.

Increase heat to medium, add the cilantro and stir for 30 seconds or until fragrant. Sprinkle with arrowroot powder and stir for 1 minute. Gradually stir in the vegetable broth and rest of the water. Bring to a boil, reduce the heat to low and simmer, covered, for 30 minutes. Cool slightly.

While soup simmers, blend the cashews and nondairy milk in a high-powered blender. Working in batches, if necessary, add soup to cashew and milk mixture and blend until smooth and creamy. Return to pot and reheat.

Season with pepper, if desired. Garnish bowls of soup with additional cilantro leaves.

PER SERVING: CALORIES 244; PROTEIN 8g; CARBOHYDRATES 35g; TOTAL FAT 9.7g; SATURATED FAT 1.8g; SODIUM 111mg; FIBER 4.6g; BETA-CAROTENE 1,085mcg; VITAMIN C 101mg; CALCIUM 43mg; IRON 2.5mg; FOLATE 86mcg; MAGNESIUM 108mg; ZINC 1.7mg; SELENIUM 5.7mcg

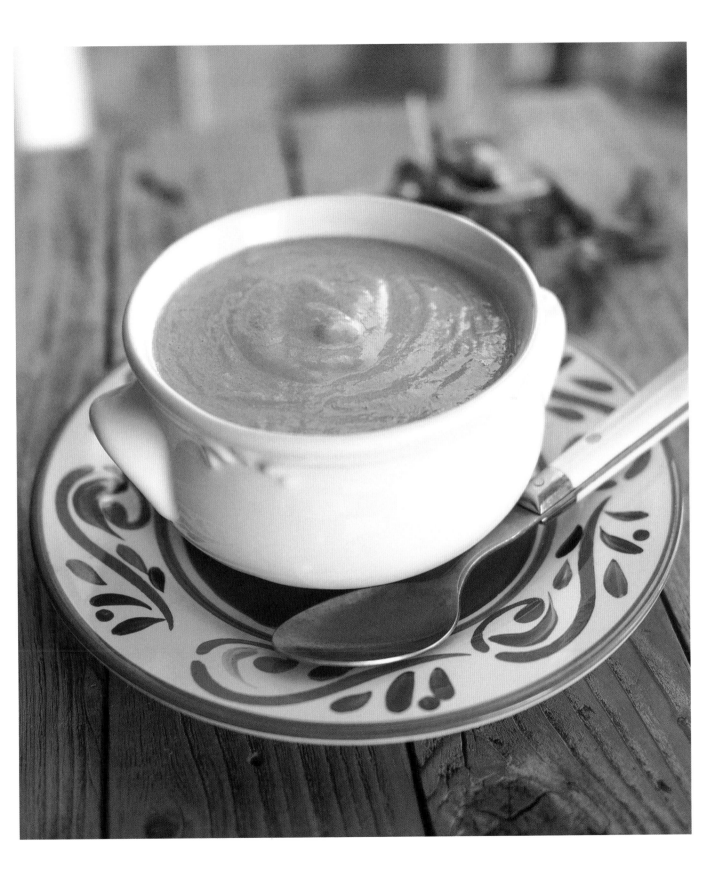

Sweet Potato Soup with Ginger and Kale

SERVES 6

1 large onion, chopped

1 tablespoon peeled and minced fresh ginger

2 pounds sweet potatoes, peeled and chopped (about 4 large or 6 medium potatoes)

5 cups low-sodium or no-salt-added vegetable broth

1 ½ cups cooked or 1 (15-ounce) can low-sodium or no-salt-added cannellini beans

¼ teaspoon black pepper

6 cups baby kale or spinach

¼ cup pumpkin seeds, toasted

Heat 2–3 tablespoons water in a large soup pot and water-sauté onion 2–3 minutes, until starting to soften. Add ginger and cook for an additional minute.

Add sweet potatoes, broth, beans, and black pepper and bring to a boil. Reduce heat, cover, and simmer for 25 minutes or until potatoes are soft.

Working in batches, blend soup and return to pot. Return to a simmer, add baby kale or spinach, and heat until wilted.

Serve in bowls and top with toasted pumpkin seeds.

PER SERVING: CALORIES 277; PROTEIN 11g; CARBOHYDRATES 54g; TOTAL FAT 3.1g; SATURATED FAT 0.6g; SODIUM 230mg; FIBER 9.7g; BETA-CAROTENE 19,048mcg; VITAMIN C 86mg; CALCIUM 205mg; IRON 4.5mg; FOLATE 80mcg; MAGNESIUM 119mg; ZINC 1.8mg; SELENIUM 2.7mcg

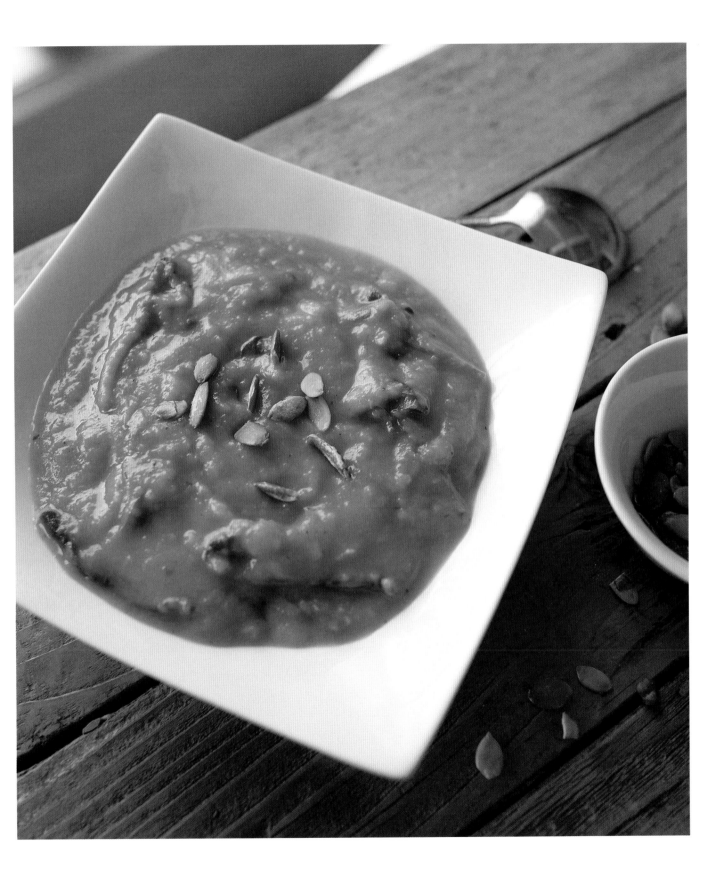

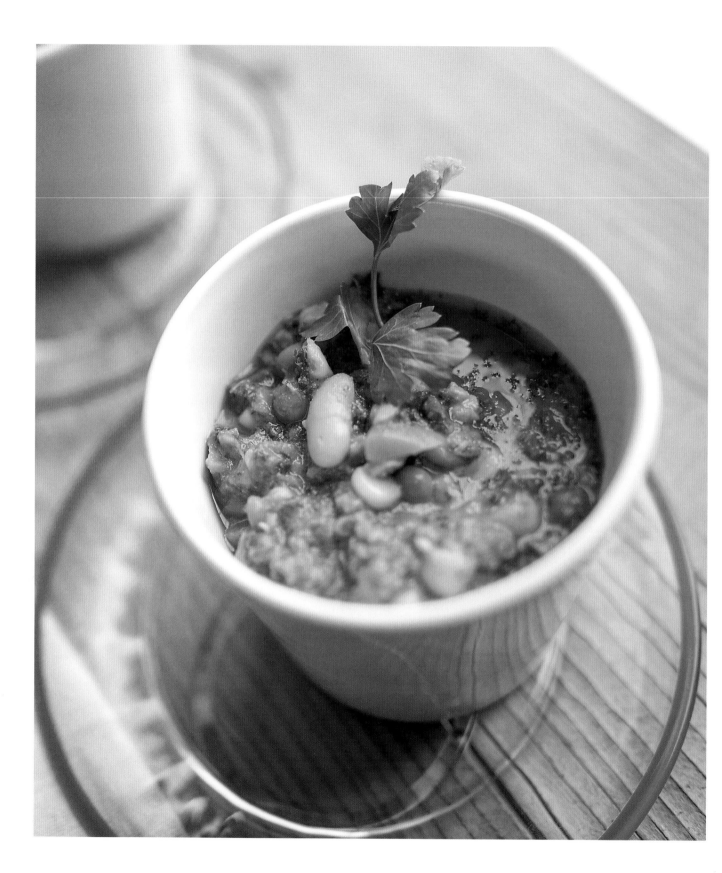

Too-Busy-to-Cook Vegetable Bean Soup

Blend 1 ½ cups of the frozen corn with the nondairy milk. Pour into a large pot. Add remaining ingredients and bring to a boil.

Reduce heat, cover, and simmer for 35 minutes. Serve.

To make an extra creamy version of this recipe, blend half of the cooked soup in a blender until creamy and add back to the pot.

SERVES 6

3 cups frozen corn, divided

2 cups unsweetened soy, hemp, or almond milk

4 cups frozen chopped kale

2 cups frozen chopped broccoli

2 cups frozen Oriental vegetables

2 cups carrot juice or 2 pounds carrots, juiced

3 cups cooked or 2 (15-ounce) cans low-sodium or no-salt-added beans

No-salt seasoning blend, adjusted to taste, or 2 tablespoons VegiZest

PER SERVING: CALORIES 301; PROTEIN 21g; CARBOHYDRATES 58g; TOTAL FAT 3.9g; SATURATED FAT 0.5g; SODIUM 154mg; FIBER 7.6g; BETA-CAROTENE 7,669mcg; VITAMIN C 98mg; CALCIUM 288mg; IRON 5.9mg; FOLATE 248mcg; MAGNESIUM 232mg; ZINC 2.7mg; SELENIUM 4.2mcg

Two-Bean Chili

1 cup chopped onion, fresh or frozen

½ cup chopped green bell pepper, fresh or frozen

1 clove garlic, chopped

¾ cup water

2 tablespoons tomato paste*

1 tablespoon chili powder

2 teaspoons ground cumin

¼ teaspoon black pepper

1 ½ cups cooked or 1 (15-ounce) can low-sodium or no-salt-added black beans, drained

3 cups cooked or 2 (15-ounce) cans low-sodium or no-salt-added red pinto or kidney beans, drained

2 cups low-sodium or no-salt-added vegetable broth

1 ½ cups diced tomatoes

1 cup frozen corn or frozen chopped broccoli (optional)

1 tablespoon yellow cornmeal

Look for tomato paste packaged in non-BPA containing glass jars.

Water-sauté onion and bell pepper in a soup pot until almost tender, or if using frozen, until thawed. Add garlic and cook for another minute.

Stir in water, tomato paste, chili powder, cumin, black pepper, beans, vegetable broth, diced tomatoes, and optional corn or broccoli if desired, and bring to a boil.

Reduce heat, cover, and simmer for 10 minutes.

Stir in cornmeal and cook for an additional 2 minutes.

TIP: Beans and greens are the most favorable foods for weight loss. They are also closely linked in scientific literature with protection against cancer, diabetes, and heart disease.

PER SERVING: CALORIES 317; PROTEIN 19g; CARBOHYDRATES 59g; TOTAL FAT 1.9g; SATURATED FAT 0.3g; SODIUM 119mg; FIBER 18.6g; BETA-CAROTENE 725mcg; VITAMIN C 31mg; CALCIUM 107mg; IRON 7.2mg; FOLATE 290mcg; MAGNESIUM 132mg; ZINC 2.6mg; SELENIUM 3.9mcg

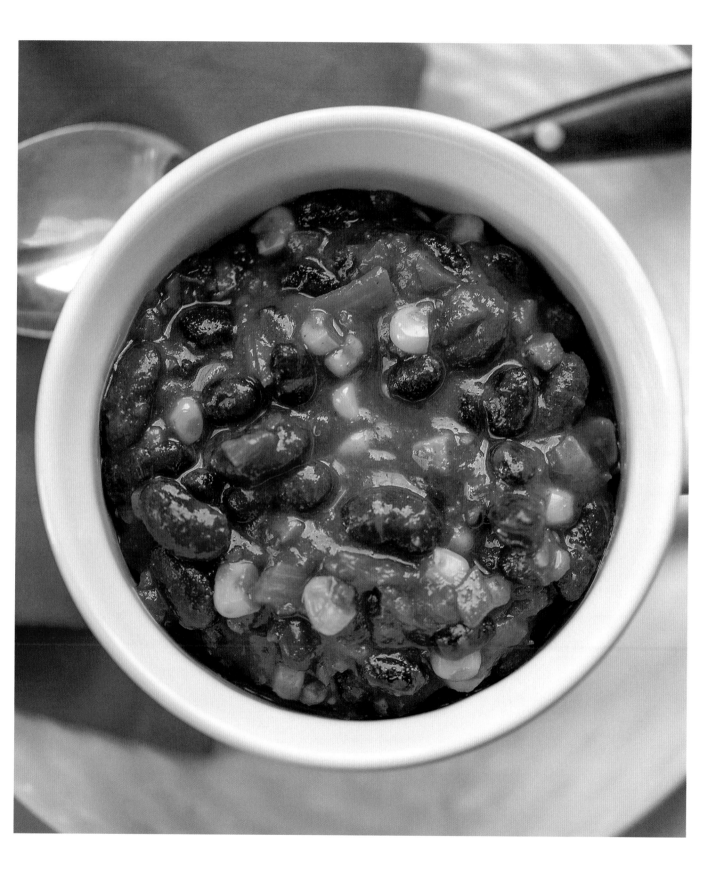

MAIN DISHES

Eating large portions of healthy food, prepared deliciously, effectively blunts your appetite for more concentrated calories and unhealthful food choices.

These main dish recipes are not only delicious and satisfying, but also very easy to prepare. Once you have mastered the basics of high-nutrient food preparation outlined in this book, such as water-sautéing and using a wok, you'll find that Nutritarian meal prep has become second nature to you. In many cases, you'll be able to put together a healthful gourmet meal in less time than it takes to get takeout!

I encourage you to follow the recipes as written until you are used to cooking Nutritarian dishes, but once you're comfortable with the techniques and familiar with the taste profiles, don't be afraid to swap vegetables and seasonings around to customize recipes to your own taste. You can also use these recipes as a starting point to create your own unique dishes.

I have included a wide range of flavors—of Italian, Asian, Indian, and Mexican origins—in the recipe selection. Some recipes use intact whole grains, and others incorporate small amounts of animal products. All are packed with flavor and are high in important nutrients.

If you would like to create your own recipe based on the Nutritarian protocols, here are some ingredient and seasoning combinations to get you started.

Choose Your Ingredients

ITALIAN	MEXICAN	ASIAN	INDIAN	GREEK	MOROCCAN
Tomatoes	Corn	Bok choy	Cauliflower	Eggplant	Tomatoes
White beans	Tomatoes	Broccoli	Lentils	Zucchini	Chickpeas
Bell peppers	Kidney beans	Snow peas	Tomatoes	White beans	Leafy greens
Zucchini	Bell peppers	String beans	Green peas	Spinach	Carrots
Leafy greens	Chili peppers	Tofu	Spinach	Tomatoes	Eggplant
Eggplant	Jicama	Cabbage	Chili peppers	Bell peppers	Onions
Onions	Onions	Mushrooms	Mushrooms	Cucumbers	Sweet potatoes
Mushrooms	Avocado	Peas	Carrots	Onions	
	Squash	Scallions			

Choose Your Seasonings

ITALIAN	MEXICAN	ASIAN	INDIAN	GREEK	MOROCCAN
Lemon	Lime	Lime	Lemon	Lemon	Lemon
Garlic	Chili powder	Ginger	Turmeric	Garlic	Cinnamon
Oregano	Cumin	Garlic	Cumin	Mint	Cumin
Basil	Cinnamon	Sesame seeds	Ginger	Dill	Garlic
Parsley	Cilantro	Vinegar	Curry powder	Parsley	Cilantro
Thyme	Cayenne pepper	Mint	Garam masala	Oregano	Raisins or currants
Marjoram	Pumpkin seeds	Bragg Liquid Aminos	Garlic	Walnuts	Black pepper
Pine nuts			Cloves		Mint

Quick and Easy Artichoke and Tomato Sauce Dinner

Heat artichoke hearts in microwave oven according to package directions; set aside.

Microwave whole garlic cloves for 1 minute. Let cool enough so you can mince them by hand or use food processor.

Place heated artichoke hearts on a microwavable plate or bowl, cover with tomato sauce, then place minced garlic on top of sauce. Heat in microwave oven until evenly heated.

SERVES 2

1 (12-ounce) box frozen artichoke hearts (no salt or seasonings added)

6–8 cloves garlic, skins removed

1 cup no-salt-added or low-sodium tomato sauce

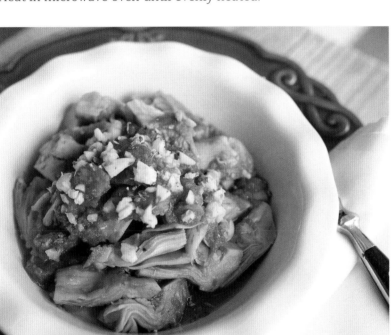

PER SERVING: CALORIES 107; PROTEIN 6g; CARBOHYDRATES 23g; TOTAL FAT 0.9g; SATURATED FAT 0.2g; SODIUM 79mg; FIBER 7.6g; BETA-CAROTENE 326mcg; VITAMIN C 18mg; CALCIUM 63mg; IRON 2.1mg; FOLATE 157mcg; MAGNESIUM 60mg; ZINC 0.8mg; SELENIUM 2.2mcg

Breaded Eggplant with Peppers

SERVES 3

1 cup (100% whole grain) bread crumbs

2 tablespoons unfortified nutritional yeast

½ teaspoon salt-free Italian seasoning

1 eggplant, peeled and sliced into ¼-inch slices

1 cup soy, hemp, or almond milk

1 red or green bell pepper, sliced

3 small cloves garlic, minced

1 ½ cups no-salt-added tomato-based pasta sauce

Preheat oven to 375°F. Lightly wipe cooking sheet with olive oil.

Combine bread crumbs, unfortified nutritional yeast, and seasoning. Dip eggplant slices into nondairy milk and then into bread crumb mixture. Place on cookie sheet. Bake 40 minutes, turning after 15–20 minutes, before bottoms start to brown.

In a large pan, water-sauté bell pepper and garlic until pepper is tender. Stir in pasta sauce.

Arrange eggplant slices on a serving plate and top with sauce.

PER SERVING: CALORIES 215; PROTEIN 10g; CARBOHYDRATES 36g; TOTAL FAT 4.1g; SATURATED FAT 0.5g; CHOLESTEROL 2.6mg; SODIUM 124mg; FIBER 10.9g; BETA-CAROTENE 1,588mcg; VITAMIN C 58mg; CALCIUM 82mg; IRON 2.7mg; FOLATE 85mcg; MAGNESIUM 78mg; ZINC 1.8mg; SELENIUM 6.3mcg

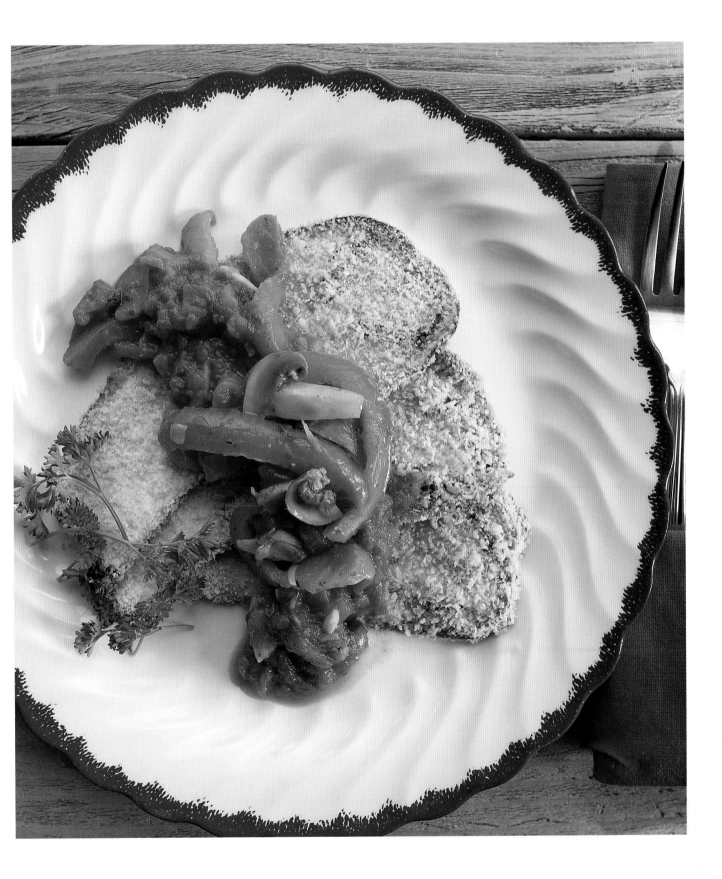

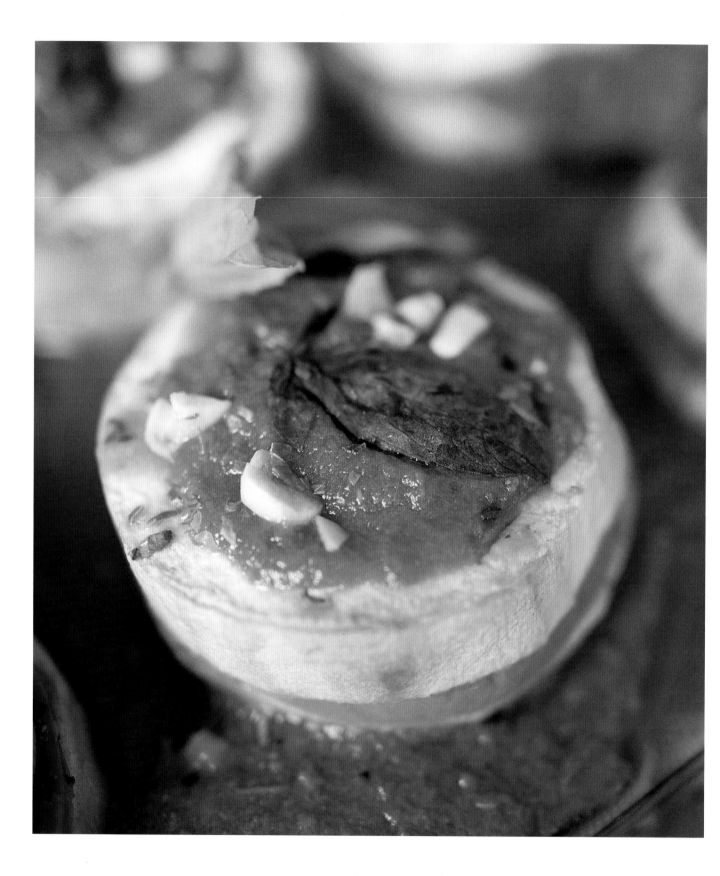

Italian Stacked Eggplant

Preheat oven to 350°F.

Cover bottom of a baking dish with pasta sauce. Place half of the eggplant slices on the sauce, top with tomato slices, and with the remaining eggplant slices. Sprinkle garlic, basil, and oregano on top.

Cover baking dish with foil and bake 30 minutes. Uncover and bake an additional 10 minutes or until eggplant is tender.

SERVES 4

½ cup no-salt-added tomato-based pasta sauce

1 medium eggplant, peeled and cut crosswise into ½-inch rounds

3 large tomatoes, sliced

5 cloves garlic, minced

3 tablespoons fresh basil leaves, rolled and sliced

½ teaspoon dried oregano

TIP: Lycopene is the signature carotenoid of the tomato. It is known for its anticancer properties, but it also has beneficial cardiovascular effects.

PER SERVING: CALORIES 134; PROTEIN 5g; CARBOHYDRATES 28g; TOTAL FAT 1.8g; SATURATED FAT 0.3g; CHOLESTEROL 1.3mg; SODIUM 35mg; FIBER 11.6g; BETA-CAROTENE 1,245mcg; VITAMIN C 35mg; CALCIUM 84mg; IRON 2mg; FOLATE 90mcg; MAGNESIUM 70mg; ZINC 0.9mg; SELENIUM 2.5mcg

Easy Ratatouille

SERVES 4

26 ounces no-salt-added crushed tomatoes

6 medium zucchini, cut into ½-inch rounds

1 large eggplant, peeled and cut into 1-inch cubes

1 onion, chopped

6 cloves garlic, minced or pressed

No-salt seasoning blend, adjusted to taste, or 2 tablespoons MatoZest

2 teaspoons fresh thyme, chopped, or 1 teaspoon dried

1 teaspoon fresh rosemary, chopped, or ½ teaspoon dried

This classic dish originated in the Provence region of France. It can be served warm or cold, as a main course or side dish, or even for breakfast.

Combine all ingredients in a large saucepan; cover and slowly simmer for 15–20 minutes or until vegetables are tender, stirring occasionally. The tomatoes and vegetables will make their own sauce.

PER SERVING: CALORIES 169; PROTEIN 9g; CARBOHYDRATES 36g; TOTAL FAT 1.9g; SATURATED FAT 0.4g; SODIUM 279mg; FIBER 11.5g; BETA-CAROTENE 621mcg; VITAMIN C 79mg; CALCIUM 152mg; IRON 4.5mg; FOLATE 141mcg; MAGNESIUM 119mg; ZINC 1.8mg; SELENIUM 3.1mcg

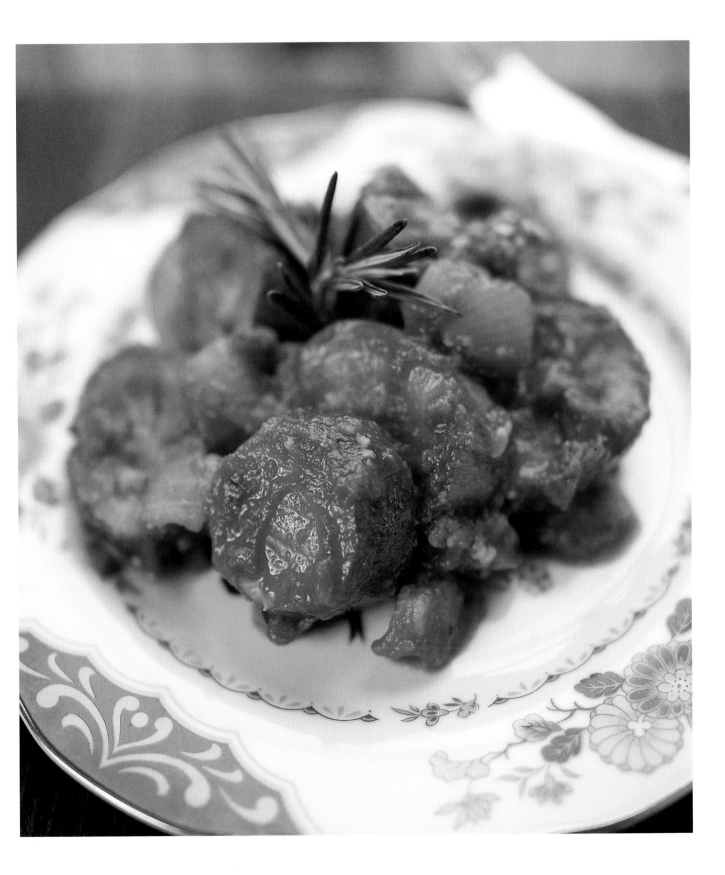

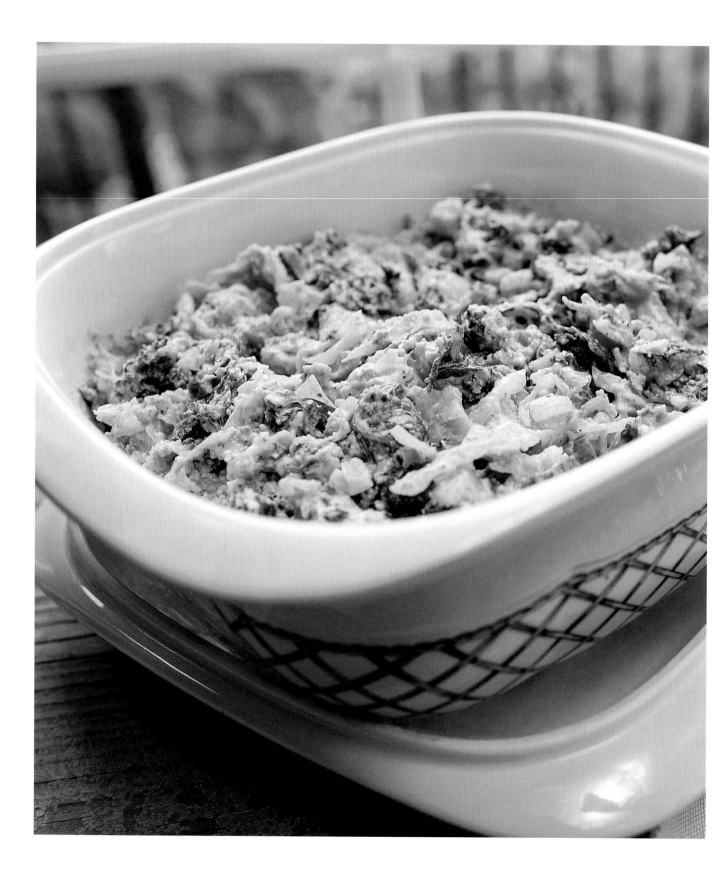

Baked Kale and Cabbage Casserole

If you will be in a rush right before dinner, assemble this casserole ahead of time and heat just before serving.

Preheat oven to 350°F.

Place ¼ cup water, onions, and Liquid Aminos in large pot. Simmer until the onion is soft, about 3 minutes. Add cabbage, kale, and carrots; cover and simmer about 12 minutes or until vegetables are tender, adding more water if necessary. Set aside.

In a high-powered blender, combine tofu, nondairy milk, unfortified nutritional yeast, basil, oregano, paprika, garlic, and almonds. Combine with vegetables and place in a baking dish.

Bake about 15 minutes or until heated through and the top is slightly crispy.

SERVES 6

2 medium onions, diced

1 teaspoon Bragg Liquid Aminos

½ head cabbage, chopped

1 bunch kale

2 carrots, peeled and diced

7 ounces silken tofu

¼ cup soy, hemp, or almond milk

¼ cup unfortified nutritional yeast

2 teaspoons dried basil

1 teaspoon dried oregano

1 teaspoon paprika

3 cloves garlic

½ cup raw almonds or ¼ cup raw almond butter

TIP: Vegetables, especially green leafy vegetables, win the nutrient density prize. The concentration of vitamins, minerals, phytochemicals, and antioxidants per calorie in vegetables is the highest, by far, of any food group.

PER SERVING: CALORIES 212; PROTEIN 14g; CARBOHYDRATES 22g; TOTAL FAT 9.5g; SATURATED FAT 1g; SODIUM 101mg; FIBER 8.8g; BETA-CAROTENE 4,032mcg; VITAMIN C 87mg; CALCIUM 404mg; IRON 3.4mg; FOLATE 99mcg; MAGNESIUM 94mg; ZINC 2.5mg; SELENIUM 7.1mcg

Creamy Polenta with Mushrooms, Kale, and Chickpeas

For the vegetables

10 ounces mushrooms, any variety or a combination of different types, sliced

3 cloves garlic, chopped

1 large red onion, sliced

2 tablespoons balsamic vinegar

5 cups chopped kale, tough stems removed

1 ½ cups diced tomatoes

1 ½ cups cooked or 1 (15-ounce) can low-sodium or no-salt-added chickpeas, drained

1 cup low-sodium or no-salt-added vegetable broth

½ teaspoon dried thyme

¼ teaspoon black pepper

⅛ teaspoon cayenne pepper

For the polenta

3 cups water

1 cup cornmeal

Heat 2–3 tablespoons water in a large skillet. Add mushrooms, garlic, and onion and water-sauté 5 minutes at medium heat or until onions are tender and mushrooms have cooked down.

Add balsamic vinegar and simmer for an additional minute. Add kale and continue cooking until kale has softened.

Add tomatoes, chickpeas, vegetable broth, thyme, black pepper, and cayenne pepper.

Simmer for 10 minutes, breaking up some of the chickpeas and tomatoes with the back of a spoon.

To prepare polenta, bring water to a boil over high heat, then slowly whisk in cornmeal. When all the cornmeal is added, reduce heat to a very low simmer, cover, and continue cooking until the polenta is smooth and thick, about 10–20 minutes, stirring every 5 minutes.

Serve polenta topped with kale and chickpea mixture.

PER SERVING: CALORIES 311; PROTEIN 14g; CARBOHYDRATES 60g; TOTAL FAT 3.7g; SATURATED FAT 0.5g; SODIUM 103mg; FIBER 10.9g; BETA-CAROTENE 8,086mcg; VITAMIN C 116mg; CALCIUM 184mg; IRON 5.3mg; FOLATE 168mcg; MAGNESIUM 118mg; ZINC 2.5mg; SELENIUM 14.9mcg

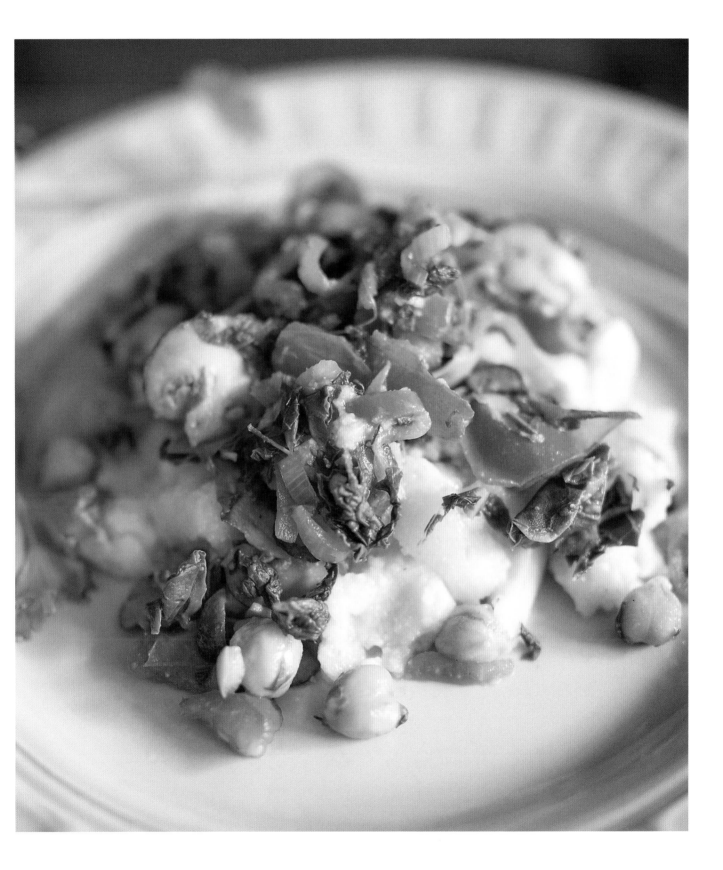

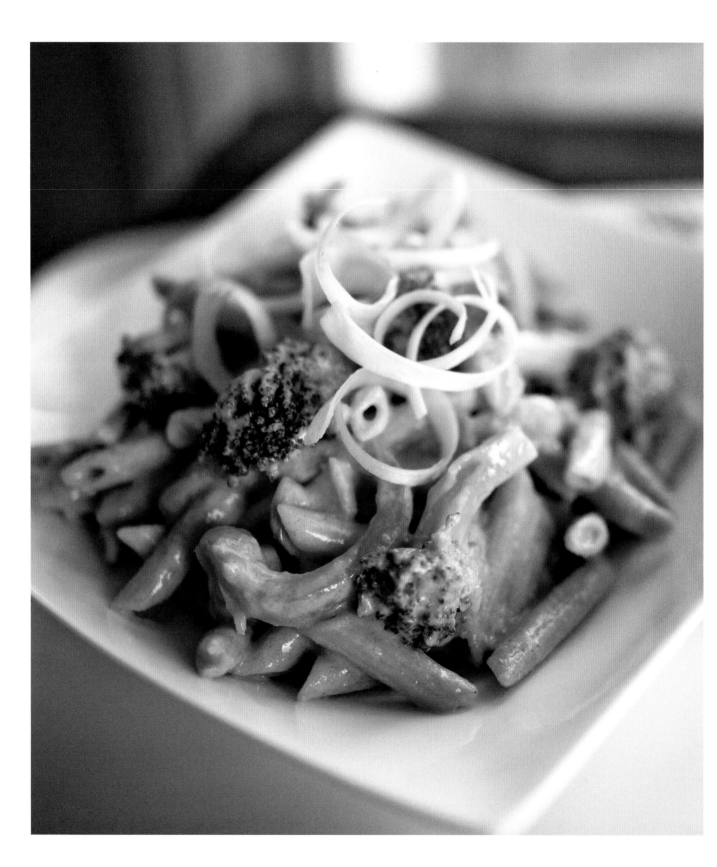

Chilled Sesame Noodles and Broccoli

In a high-powered blender, puree all of the sauce ingredients until smooth.

In a large bowl, toss the cooked pasta, steamed broccoli, red pepper, and scallions with the sauce until thoroughly coated.

Divide among six plates and serve immediately or refrigerate until ready to use.

SERVES 6

8 ounces bean pasta,* cooked according to package directions, rinsed under cold water, and drained

2 pounds fresh or frozen broccoli florets, steamed

1 large red bell pepper, or 2 roasted red peppers, diced

6 scallions, thinly sliced

For the sauce

¼ cup unhulled sesame seeds, lightly pan toasted

1 cup unsweetened almond or soy milk

6 medjool dates or 12 regular dates, pitted

½ tablespoon minced ginger

4 cloves garlic, peeled

¼ teaspoon red pepper flakes, or to taste

3 tablespoons rice vinegar

....

* Several varieties of organic bean pasta are available at www.drfuhrman.com.

PER SERVING: CALORIES 281; PROTEIN 17g; CARBOHYDRATES 47g; TOTAL FAT 4.6g; SATURATED FAT 0.5g; SODIUM 71mg; FIBER 13.1g; BETA-CAROTENE 1,096mcg; VITAMIN C 173mg; CALCIUM 308mg; IRON 6.2mg; FOLATE 142mcg; MAGNESIUM 69mg; ZINC 3mg; SELENIUM 6.3mcg

Chipotle Beans and Greens

SERVES 6

1 ½ pounds fresh collard greens, tough stems removed, chopped

3 (15-ounce) cans (about 4 ½ cups) low-sodium or no-salt-added diced tomatoes*

4 ounces no-salt-added tomato paste*

6 cups cooked or 4 (15-ounce) cans no-salt-added or low-sodium pinto beans, drained

1 teaspoon garlic powder

¼ teaspoon chipotle chili powder, or more to taste

....

Choose tomato products packaged in cartons or glass. These materials do not contain BPA.

In a large pot, water-sauté collard greens until almost tender, about 3 minutes. Stir in remaining ingredients. Mix well and simmer for 10 minutes.

This is good when stored in the refrigerator overnight and reheated.

PER SERVING: CALORIES 292; PROTEIN 17g; CARBOHYDRATES 62g; TOTAL FAT 1.6g; SATURATED FAT 0.3g; SODIUM 1,587mg; FIBER 16.6g; BETA-CAROTENE 3,333mcg; VITAMIN C 64mg; CALCIUM 163mg; IRON 8mg; FOLATE 207mcg; MAGNESIUM 130mg; ZINC 2.1mg; SELENIUM 16.4mcg

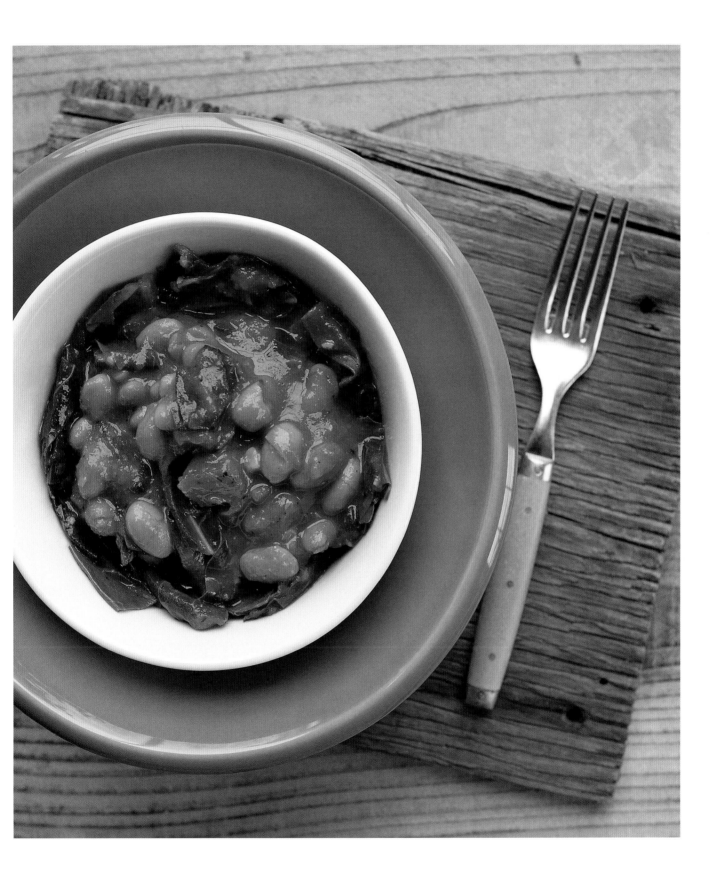

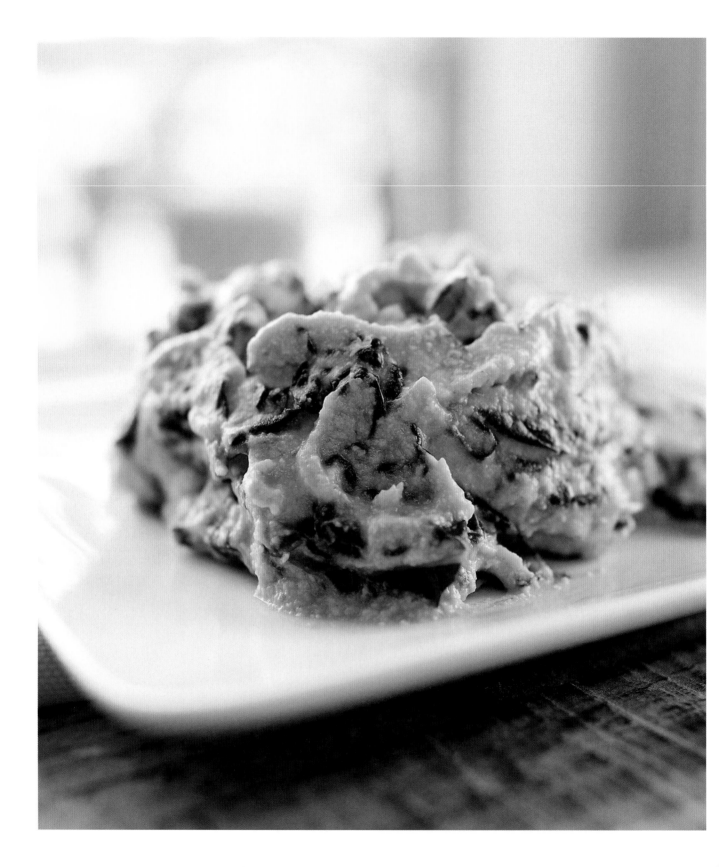

"Creamed" Kale and Sweet Potatoes

Place kale in a steamer pot. Steam 8 minutes or until soft.

Meanwhile, place remaining ingredients in a high-powered blender and blend until very smooth.

Place kale in a strainer and press to remove excess water.

In a bowl, mix kale with cream sauce.

SERVES 4

2 bunches kale, tough stems and center ribs removed, chopped

1 cup raw cashews

1 cup unsweetened soy, hemp, or almond milk

1 cup cooked, diced sweet potatoes*

1 clove garlic, chopped

¼ cup chopped shallots

½ tablespoon apple cider vinegar

No-salt seasoning blend, adjusted to taste, or 1 tablespoon VegiZest

Pinch of nutmeg

To cook sweet potatoes, pierce whole potato in several spots with a fork. Bake at 350°F for 50 minutes or until soft, or microwave on high for 12–16 minutes. Let potato cool; remove skin and dice.

TIP: Low-nutrient eating drives overeating behavior and food cravings. A properly nourished body, however, is satisfied with the right number of calories and will naturally gravitate toward its ideal weight.

PER SERVING: CALORIES 301; PROTEIN 12g; CARBOHYDRATES 31g; TOTAL FAT 16.6g; SATURATED FAT 2.9g; SODIUM 89mg; FIBER 4.5g; BETA-CAROTENE 9,370mcg; VITAMIN C 88mg; CALCIUM 147mg; IRON 4.5mg; FOLATE 55mcg; MAGNESIUM 154mg; ZINC 2.5mg; SELENIUM 10.9mcg

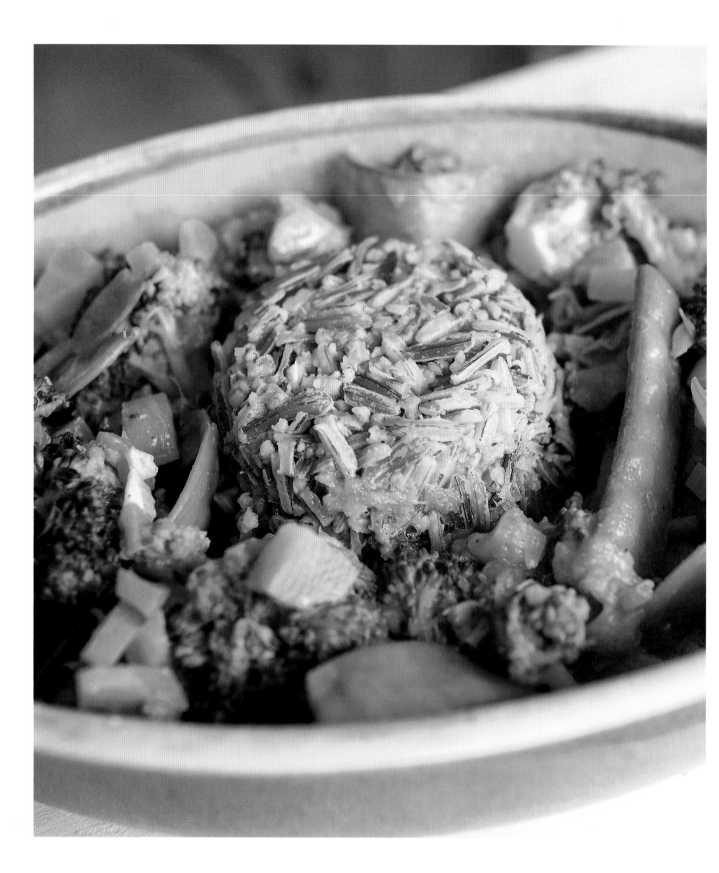

Coconut Curry with Broccoli and Snow Peas

Heat ¼ cup water in a large soup pot and add onion, garlic, ginger, carrots, and black pepper. Water-sauté for 5 minutes or until vegetables start to soften.

Add broccoli, tomatoes, vegetable broth, curry powder, and cayenne pepper; bring to a boil, reduce heat, cover, and simmer 10 minutes.

Add coconut milk, lime juice, and snow peas; return to a simmer, cover, and cook for an additional 5 minutes.

Serve over quinoa, wild rice, farro, or whole grain.

SERVES 4

1 medium onion, chopped

4 cloves garlic, minced

1 tablespoon fresh ginger, minced

½ cup diced carrots

¼ teaspoon ground black pepper

6 cups broccoli florets

1 ½ cups low-sodium or no-salt-added packaged diced tomatoes*

2 cups low-sodium or no-salt-added vegetable broth

1 tablespoon curry powder

⅛ teaspoon ground cayenne pepper, or to taste

1 ½ cups light coconut milk

1 tablespoon lime juice

6 ounces snow peas, trimmed

4 cups cooked whole grain such as quinoa, wild rice, or farro

Choose tomato products packaged in BPA-free cartons.

PER SERVING: CALORIES 363; PROTEIN 13g; CARBOHYDRATES 53g; TOTAL FAT 12.7g; SATURATED FAT 8.4g; SODIUM 147mg; FIBER 10.6g; BETA-CAROTENE 2,351mcg; VITAMIN C 162mg; CALCIUM 158mg; IRON 6.4mg; FOLATE 189mcg; MAGNESIUM 165mg; ZINC 2.7mg; SELENIUM 4.6mcg

Curried Chickpeas and Sweet Potatoes

SERVES 5

6 cups sweet potatoes, peeled and diced

⅓ cup water or low-sodium vegetable broth

2 teaspoons VegiZest or other no-salt seasoning, adjusted to taste

1 large onion, diced

1 tablespoon fresh ginger, minced

3 cloves garlic, minced or pressed

2 large red bell peppers, diced

2 tablespoons curry powder

3 cups cooked or 2 (15-ounce) cans low-sodium or no-salt-added chickpeas, drained

1 tablespoon apple cider vinegar

Place sweet potatoes in a large saucepan filled with 1 inch water and fitted with a steamer basket; steam for 10 minutes or until cooked through. Set aside and keep warm.

In another large pot, heat ⅓ cup water and stir in VegiZest, onion, ginger, garlic, red peppers, and curry powder. Stir, cover, and cook for 3–5 minutes or until vegetables are tender. Add chickpeas and simmer uncovered for 5 minutes.

Add vinegar and sweet potatoes and heat for a few more minutes, stirring gently. Add additional water or vegetable broth if needed to adjust consistency.

PER SERVING: CALORIES 352; PROTEIN 13g; CARBOHYDRATES 70g; TOTAL FAT 3.3g; SATURATED FAT 0.4g; SODIUM 113mg; FIBER 15.5g; BETA-CAROTENE 14,749mcg; VITAMIN C 95mg; CALCIUM 138mg; IRON 5.3mg; FOLATE 238mcg; MAGNESIUM 110mg; ZINC 2.4mg; SELENIUM 5.7mcg

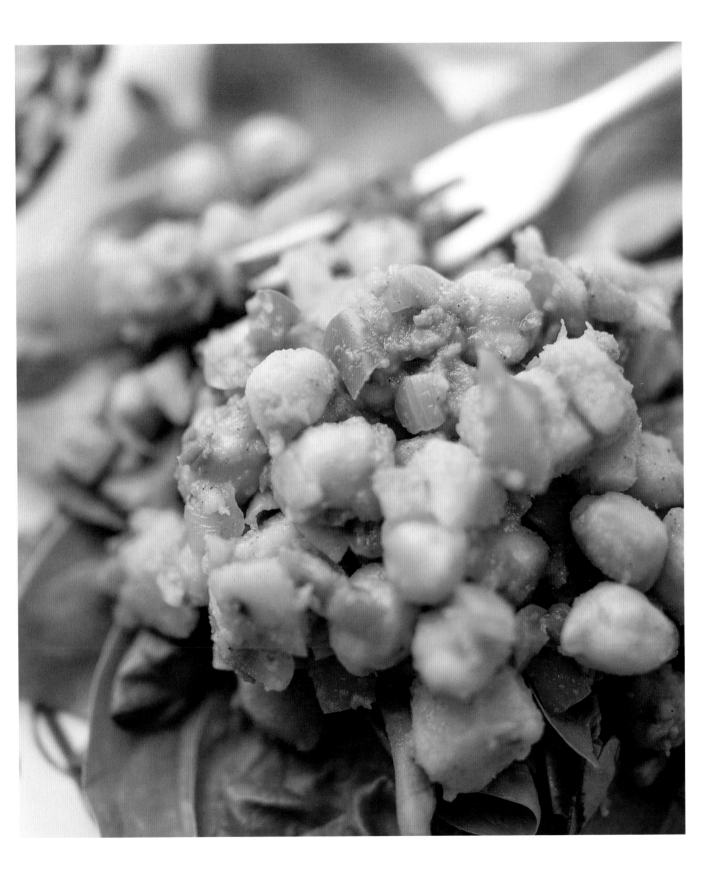

Lemon Herb Cauliflower Rice

SERVES 4

1 head cauliflower, cut into florets

2 cloves garlic, chopped

2 tablespoons lemon juice

¼ cup chopped fresh basil, dill, or parsley

¼ cup chopped almonds and/or raisins (optional)

Grate cauliflower or pulse in a food processor until it resembles rice.

Add 2 tablespoons water and "riced" cauliflower to a skillet. Cook for 8 minutes. Add garlic and cook for an additional 2 minutes. Add additional water if needed to prevent sticking.

Remove from heat and stir in lemon juice and herbs. If desired, stir in chopped almonds and/or raisins.

PER SERVING: CALORIES 41; PROTEIN 3g; CARBOHYDRATES 8g; TOTAL FAT 0.5g; SATURATED FAT 0.1g; SODIUM 45mg; FIBER 3g; BETA-CAROTENE 83mcg; VITAMIN C 75mg; CALCIUM 40mg; IRON 0.7mg; FOLATE 87mcg; MAGNESIUM 25mg; ZINC 0.4mg; SELENIUM 1.1mcg

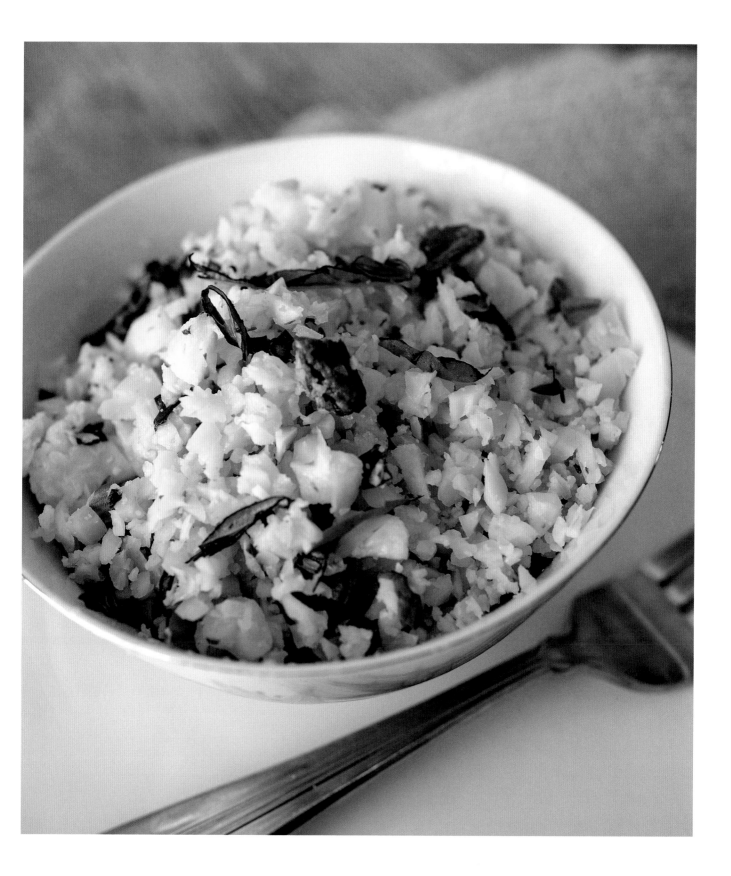

Mashed Cauliflower and Brussels Sprouts

SERVES 4

1 onion, chopped

1 head cauliflower, cut into large pieces

1 pound Brussels sprouts, cut in half

½ cup walnuts

1 teaspoon no-salt seasoning blend, adjusted to taste

Soy, hemp, or almond milk, as needed to adjust consistency

Because cruciferous vegetables contain compounds that have powerful protective effects against many cancers, you should strive to have one or two servings daily. This combo of cauliflower and Brussels sprouts is one delicious way to accomplish that goal.

Sauté onion in a little water until translucent and starting to soften. Add cauliflower and Brussels sprouts, cover and steam until tender, about 10 minutes, adding water as needed to prevent sticking.

Place in a high-powered blender with walnuts and seasoning and puree until creamy.

Add a little nondairy milk as needed to thin—the mixture should be the consistency of mashed potatoes.

PER SERVING: CALORIES 182; PROTEIN 9g; CARBOHYDRATES 22g; TOTAL FAT 9.1g; SATURATED FAT 1g; SODIUM 77mg; FIBER 8.8g; BETA-CAROTENE 517mcg; VITAMIN C 169mg; CALCIUM 115mg; IRON 2.8mg; FOLATE 172mcg; MAGNESIUM 73mg; ZINC 1.3mg; SELENIUM 3.5mcg

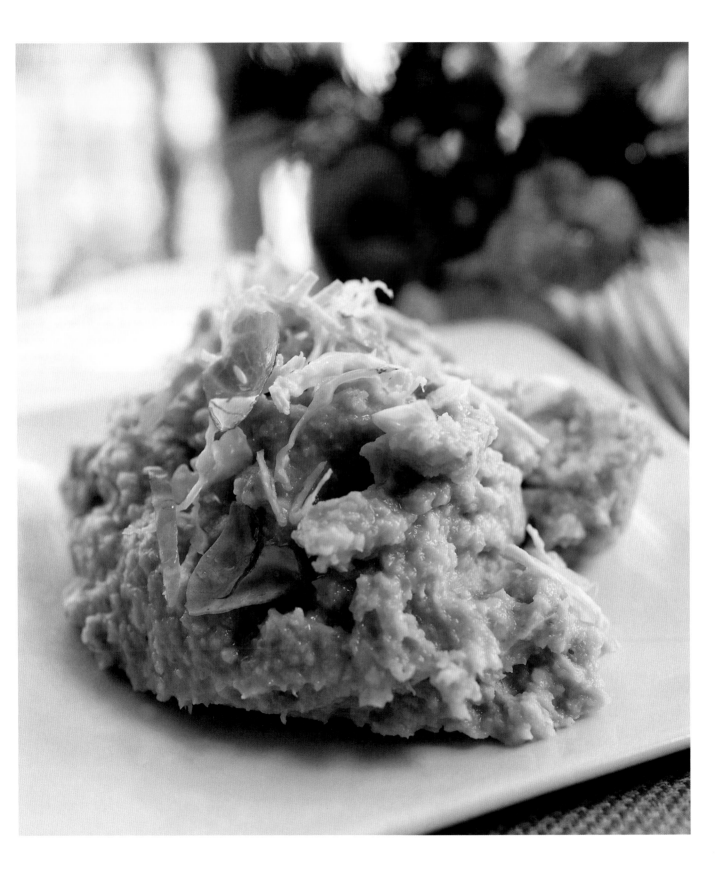

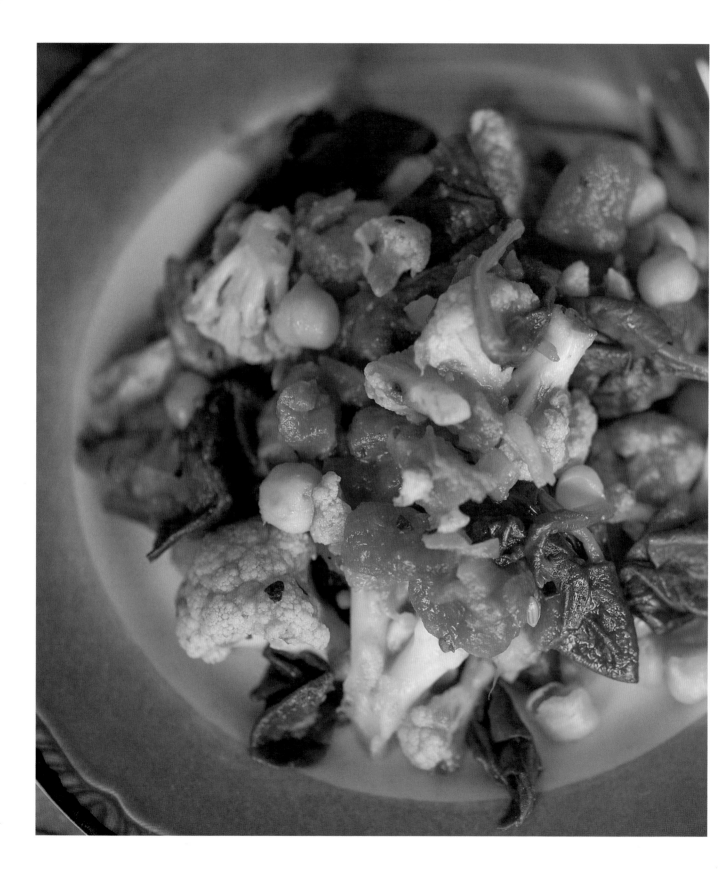

Roasted Cauliflower with Chickpeas, Tomatoes, and Spinach

Preheat oven to 400°F.

Place cauliflower on a lightly oiled baking pan and bake 20 minutes or until cauliflower is tender, stirring frequently.

Heat 2–3 tablespoons water in a large sauté pan and water-sauté onions until they start to soften. Add garlic, fennel seeds, cumin, and black and cayenne pepper; continue to cook for 1 minute, adding more water as needed.

Add tomatoes, chickpeas, roasted cauliflower, and ½ cup water; bring to a boil.

Reduce heat and simmer until liquid has slightly thickened, about 15 minutes. Fold in spinach and cook until just wilted, about 1–2 minutes.

If desired, serve on top of a whole grain.

SERVES 4

1 head cauliflower, cored and cut into small florets

1 medium onion, chopped

2 cloves garlic, minced

1 teaspoon fennel seeds

1 ½ teaspoons ground cumin

¼ teaspoon black pepper

Pinch of ground cayenne pepper, or more to taste

26 ounces packaged chopped tomatoes*

1 ½ cups cooked or 1 (15-ounce) can low-sodium or no-salt-added chickpeas, drained

1 (5-ounce) package fresh baby spinach or baby kale

Whole grain such as polenta, quinoa, farro, or wild rice (optional)

Choose tomato products packed in non-BPA cartons.

PER SERVING: CALORIES 197; PROTEIN 12g; CARBOHYDRATES 36g; TOTAL FAT 2.8g; SATURATED FAT 0.4g; SODIUM 89mg; FIBER 11.4g; BETA-CAROTENE 2,850mcg; VITAMIN C 110mg; CALCIUM 139mg; IRON 4.6mg; FOLATE 291mcg; MAGNESIUM 108mg; ZINC 2mg; SELENIUM 3.9mcg

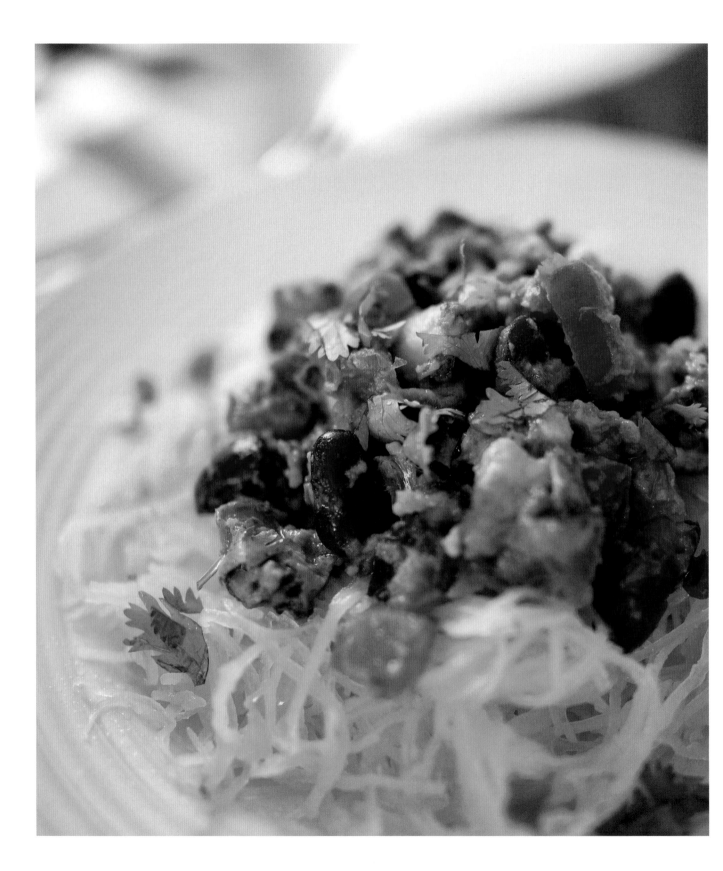

Mexican-Style Spaghetti Squash with Guacamole

Preheat oven to 350°F.

Place squash on a baking sheet, cut side facing down. Bake 45–50 minutes, until flesh is tender when pierced with a fork and easily comes apart.

While the squash is baking, make the guacamole. Using a fork, mash the avocados in a medium bowl. Add the onions, tomatoes, beans, garlic, lime juice, cumin, cilantro, and red pepper flakes and mix well.

Use a fork to separate the flesh from the shell of the squash and shred into spaghetti-like strands. Season with cumin and chili powder. Serve the spaghetti squash topped with a dollop of guacamole.

SERVES 3

For the spaghetti squash

1 large spaghetti squash, sliced in half lengthwise, seeds removed

¼ teaspoon ground cumin

¼ teaspoon ground chili powder

For the guacamole

2 ripe avocados, peeled and pitted

¼ cup chopped onions

⅔ cup chopped plum tomatoes

1 ½ cups cooked or 1 (15-ounce) can low-sodium or no-salt-added red kidney beans, drained

1 clove garlic, minced

1 tablespoon fresh lime juice

½ teaspoon ground cumin

¼ cup chopped cilantro

Red pepper flakes, to taste

PER SERVING: CALORIES 366; PROTEIN 12g; CARBOHYDRATES 52g; TOTAL FAT 15.5g; SATURATED FAT 2.2g; SODIUM 73mg; FIBER 18g; BETA-CAROTENE 511mcg; VITAMIN C 29mg; CALCIUM 118mg; IRON 4.8mg; FOLATE 231mcg; MAGNESIUM 109mg; ZINC 2.3mg; SELENIUM 2.7mcg

Mushroom Kale Bean Pasta

SERVES 4

8 ounces bean fettuccini*

1 shallot, finely chopped

1 clove fresh garlic, minced

2 cups mushrooms, sliced (preferably shiitake, maitake, or oyster mushrooms)

10 grape tomatoes, halved

1 teaspoon dry oregano

1 teaspoon dry basil

2 tablespoons unfortified nutritional yeast

2 tablespoons unflavored soy, hemp, or almond milk

2 cups baby kale, chopped

¼ teaspoon dried red pepper flakes

Several varieties of bean pasta are available at www.drfuhrman .com.

Finding a dish that is healthful as well as indulgent is not too much to ask. Enjoy this pasta recipe without a trace of guilt.

Cook bean pasta according to package instructions; drain and set aside.

In the same pot, heat 1–2 tablespoons water over medium heat. Add shallot and garlic and water-sauté 1–2 minutes. Add sliced mushrooms and sauté for 4 minutes or until mushrooms soften and liquid is evaporated.

With the heat on low, add tomatoes, oregano, basil, and cooked bean fettuccine.

Stir unfortified nutritional yeast and nondairy milk together and add to pot. Cover and heat through for 2 minutes.

Add chopped kale; cover pot to quickly soften kale for 30 seconds. Season with hot pepper flakes.

PER SERVING: CALORIES 271; PROTEIN 20g; CARBOHYDRATES 46g; TOTAL FAT 1.7g; SATURATED FAT 0.1g; SODIUM 24mg; FIBER 12.8g; BETA-CAROTENE 3,289mcg; VITAMIN C 47mg; CALCIUM 240mg; IRON 7mg; FOLATE 53mcg; MAGNESIUM 31mg; ZINC 3.8mg; SELENIUM 4.1mcg

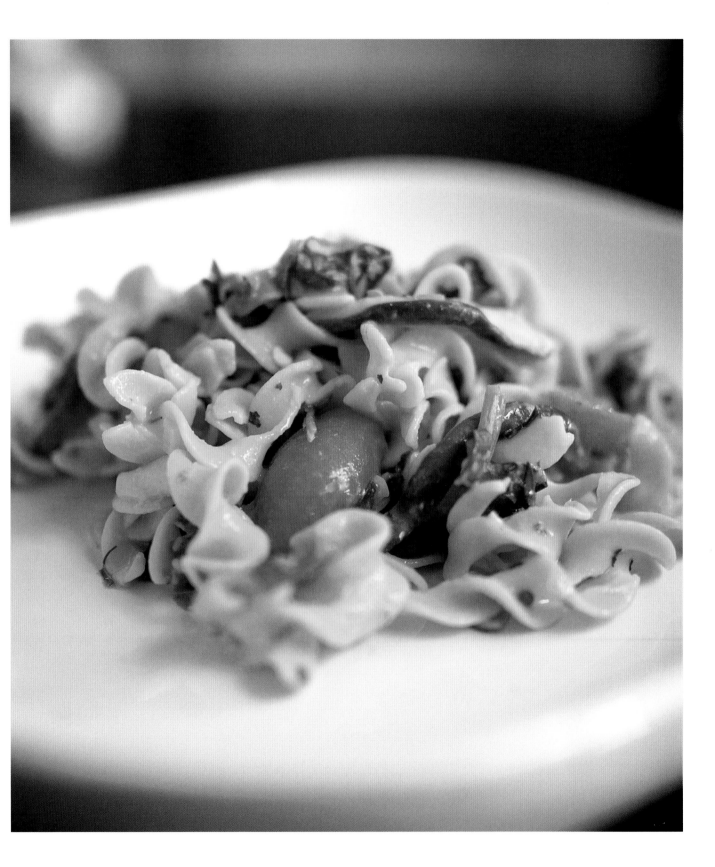

Quick Sautéed Greens, Beans, and Garlic

SERVES 2

3 cloves garlic, minced

1 large bunch (about 1 pound) greens (such as kale, collards, mustard greens, bok choy, or broccoli rabe), tough stems removed, chopped

⅛ teaspoon hot pepper flakes

1 cup (or more) low-sodium or no-salt-added vegetable broth

1 ½ cups cooked or 1 (15-ounce) can low-sodium or no-salt-added cannellini (or other) beans, drained

2 teaspoons flavored vinegar or sherry wine vinegar

No time to cook is no excuse. It takes only a few minutes to whip together a flavorful bowl of greens and beans. Kale, collards, mustard greens, bok choy, and broccoli rabe all work well in this recipe.

Heat 2–3 tablespoons water in a large skillet. Add garlic and cook for 1 minute, then add greens gradually until they are wilted. Add hot pepper flakes and vegetable broth, cover, and simmer until greens are tender, about 6–8 minutes, depending on the kind of greens you use. Add additional broth as needed.

Add beans and simmer, uncovered, until mixture is heated through and liquid is almost absorbed, about 2 minutes. Stir in vinegar.

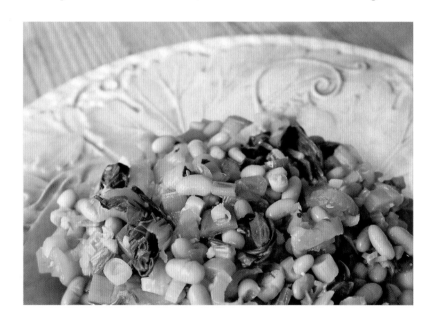

PER SERVING: CALORIES 315; PROTEIN 21g; CARBOHYDRATES 59g; TOTAL FAT 2.1g; SATURATED FAT 0.3g; SODIUM 175mg; FIBER 13.9g; BETA-CAROTENE 20,949mcg; VITAMIN C 274mg; CALCIUM 447mg; IRON 9.1mg; FOLATE 175mcg; MAGNESIUM 163mg; ZINC 2.9mg; SELENIUM 4.4mcg

Sautéed Cabbage and Onions

In a small pan over medium-low heat, toast the sesame seeds, stirring constantly, until very lightly browned, about 1 minute. Transfer to a dish and set aside.

Pour the broth into a large frying pan, bring to a boil over high heat, and cook to reduce and concentrate the broth, 2–3 minutes.

Add the onions and cabbage to the broth, reduce heat to medium, and cook, stirring constantly, until cabbage and onions are tender, about 15 minutes. The broth should be almost totally absorbed.

Stir the vinegar, toasted sesame seeds, and black pepper into the cabbage.

SERVES 4

2 tablespoons unhulled sesame seeds

1 ½ cups no-salt-added or low-sodium vegetable broth

2 medium onions, sliced

1 small head cabbage, thinly sliced lengthwise and then cut in half crosswise

2 tablespoons balsamic vinegar

¼ teaspoon black pepper, or to taste

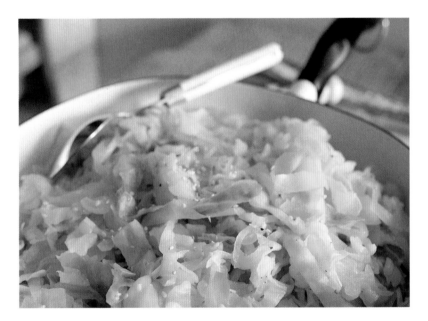

PER SERVING: CALORIES 100; PROTEIN 4g; CARBOHYDRATES 18g; TOTAL FAT 2.5g; SATURATED FAT 0.4g; SODIUM 86mg; FIBER 6g; BETA-CAROTENE 76mcg; VITAMIN C 69mg; CALCIUM 138mg; IRON 1.8mg; FOLATE 92mcg; MAGNESIUM 43mg; ZINC 0.8mg; SELENIUM 2.4mcg

Perfect Kale Sauté

SERVES 2

1 small onion, thinly sliced

1 clove garlic, chopped

¼ teaspoon crushed red pepper flakes

1 bunch kale, leaves removed from tough stems and chopped

2 carrots, shredded or sliced thin with a vegetable peeler

1 tablespoon toasted sesame seeds

In a large pan, water-sauté onion, garlic, and red pepper flakes for 1 minute.

Add half the kale, stir for 1 minute, then add remaining kale and cook until softened. Use a small amount of water as needed to prevent sticking.

Add shredded carrots and continue cooking 2–4 minutes until kale is tender.

Toss with sesame seeds.

PER SERVING: CALORIES 140; PROTEIN 7g; CARBOHYDRATES 26g; TOTAL FAT 3.2g; SATURATED FAT 0.4g; SODIUM 114mg; FIBER 6.2g; BETA-CAROTENE 19,092mcg; VITAMIN C 178mg; CALCIUM 231mg; IRON 3.1mg; FOLATE 66mcg; MAGNESIUM 75mg; ZINC 1.3mg; SELENIUM 3.1mcg

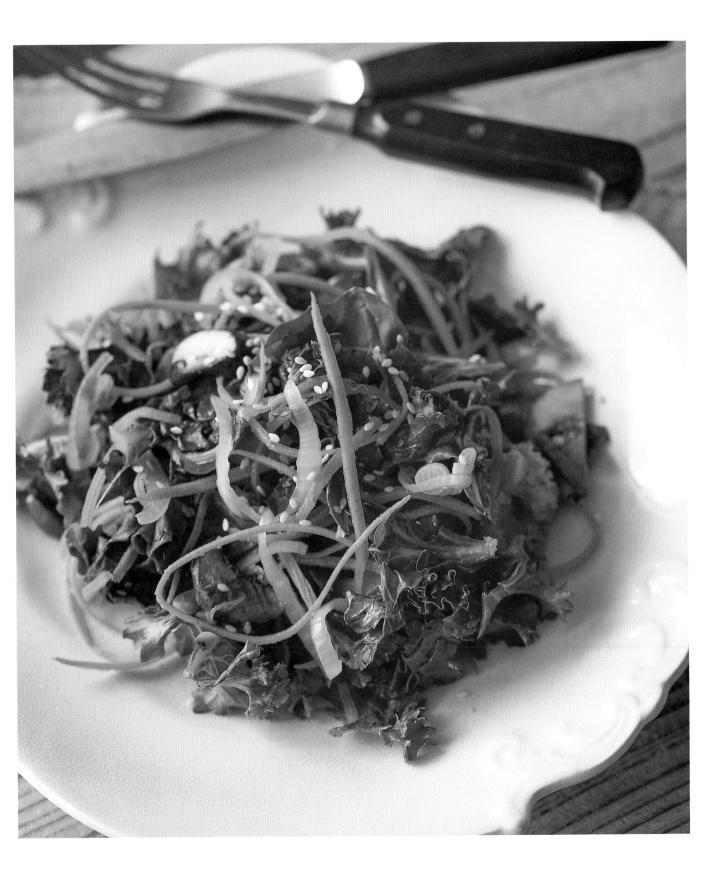

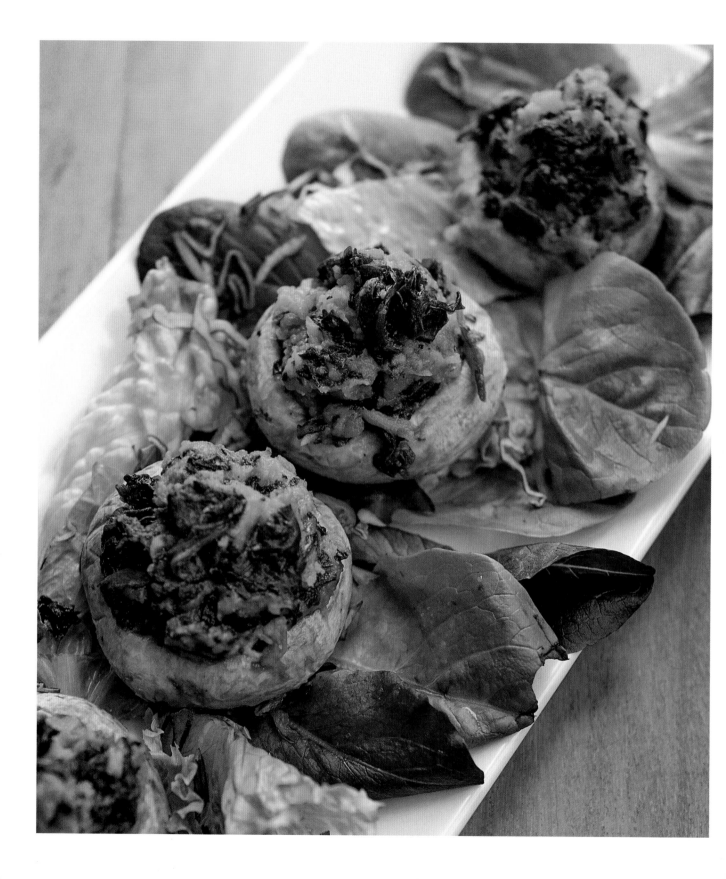

Sweet Potato Stuffed Mushrooms

Pierce sweet potato in several places with a fork. Bake at 350°F for 50 minutes or until soft, or microwave on high for 12–16 minutes. Let potato cool, remove skin, and mash.

In a large pan, heat 2–3 tablespoons water and water-sauté onion for 2 minutes; add chopped mushroom stems and garlic and continue to sauté until onions and mushrooms are tender, about 3 minutes. Add mushroom caps to pan, along with vegetable broth; bring to a simmer and cook for 5 minutes.

Remove mushroom caps from pan and place on a lightly oiled baking sheet.

Mix spinach and mashed sweet potato into onion mixture. Season with black pepper.

Fill mushroom caps with sweet potato mixture. Bake 15–20 minutes, still at 350°F, or until mushrooms are tender and filling is heated through. Drizzle with a few drops of balsamic vinegar or your favorite flavored vinegar.

SERVES 4

1 large sweet potato

1 small onion, chopped

10 ounces baby bella (or crimini) mushrooms (about 16 mushrooms), stems removed and chopped

2 cloves garlic, minced

¼ cup low-sodium or no-salt-added vegetable broth

½ cup thawed frozen spinach, liquid squeezed out

Black pepper to taste

Balsamic vinegar or flavored vinegar to taste

PER SERVING: CALORIES 73; PROTEIN 4g; CARBOHYDRATES 15g; TOTAL FAT 0.4g; SATURATED FAT 0.1g; SODIUM 44mg; FIBER 3.1g; BETA-CAROTENE 6,552mcg; VITAMIN C 13mg; CALCIUM 54mg; IRON 1.1mg; FOLATE 46mcg; MAGNESIUM 36mg; ZINC 0.7mg; SELENIUM 8.2mcg

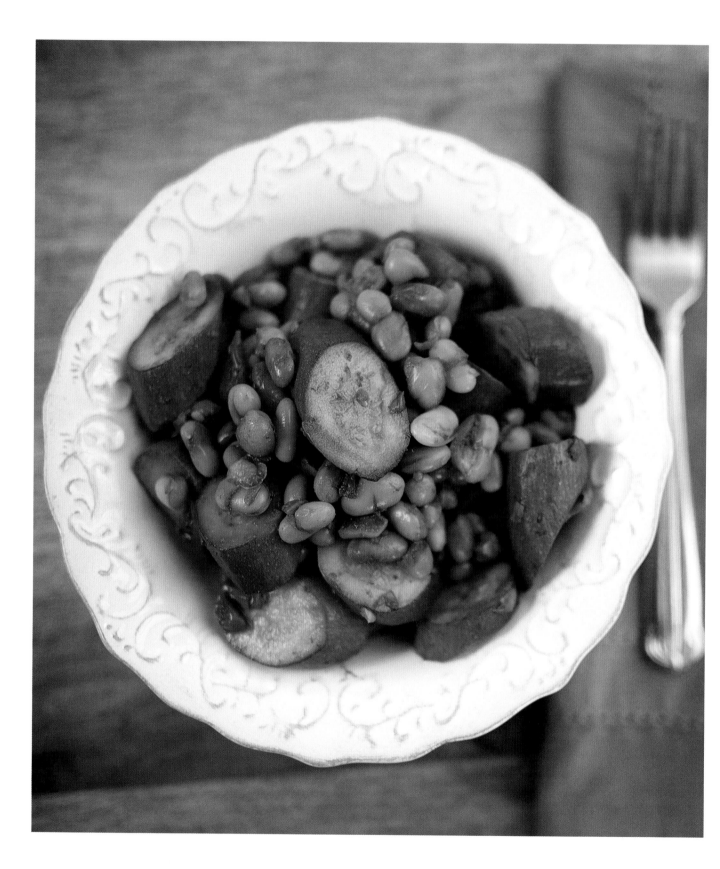

Tangy White Beans and Zucchini

Water-sauté zucchini and garlic in 2 tablespoons water over medium heat for 5 minutes, or until tender. Add beans and vinegar; cook for 5 minutes.

3 medium zucchini, cut into small chunks

2 cloves garlic, minced

1 ½ cups cooked or 1 (15-ounce) can low-sodium or no-salt-added great northern beans, drained

¼ cup balsamic vinegar

PER SERVING: CALORIES 236; PROTEIN 15g; CARBOHYDRATES 44g; TOTAL FAT 1.1g; SATURATED FAT 0.3g; SODIUM 16mg; FIBER 12.6g; BETA-CAROTENE 353mcg; VITAMIN C 53mg; CALCIUM 148mg; IRON 4.1mg; FOLATE 221mcg; MAGNESIUM 121mg; ZINC 2.1mg; SELENIUM 6.5mcg

Tofu "Meatballs"

SERVES 4

8 ounces firm tofu, drained

¼ cup ground walnuts

¼ cup old-fashioned oats, blended to make coarse crumbs

2 tablespoons whole wheat flour (or more old-fashioned oats)

1 tablespoon dried parsley flakes

¼ cup minced onion

½ teaspoon dried oregano, or to taste

½ teaspoon dried basil, or to taste

1 teaspoon Bragg Liquid Aminos or low-sodium soy sauce

These "meatballs" are surprisingly easy to make, and they bake up very nicely. Serve them topped with tomato sauce or with a side of sautéed greens.

Preheat oven to 350°F.

Mix all ingredients very well, using hands if necessary.

Form into 2-inch balls. Place on a baking pan that has been lightly oiled or lined with parchment paper. Bake for 30–35 minutes or until golden.

PER SERVING: CALORIES 106; PROTEIN 6g; CARBOHYDRATES 10g; TOTAL FAT 5.3g; SATURATED FAT 0.6g; SODIUM 78mg; FIBER 1.7g; BETA-CAROTENE 9mcg; VITAMIN C 1mg; CALCIUM 39mg; IRON 2.5mg; FOLATE 10mcg; MAGNESIUM 33mg; ZINC 0.7mg; SELENIUM 2.7mcg

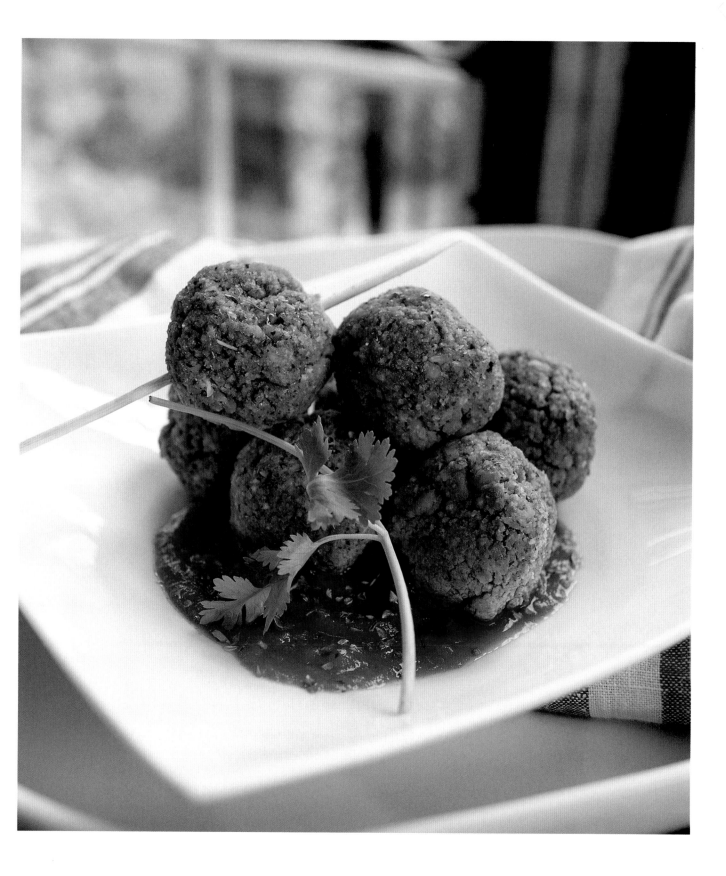

Japanese Curry Stir Fry

SERVES 6

1 cup uncooked wild rice

2 cups (10-ounce bag) frozen shelled edamame

1 large red onion, sliced

6 cups chopped baby bok choy, stems and leaves separated

16 ounces mushrooms, sliced

For the curry sauce

½ cup raw almonds or cashews

1 tablespoon tomato paste*

2 small carrots

½ apple

5 unsulfured apricot halves

2 regular dates or 1 medjool date, pitted

1 teaspoon curry powder (preferably Asian curry powder, such as S&B Oriental Curry Powder)

½ teaspoon ground turmeric

1 cup water

....

Look for tomato paste packaged in non-BPA-containing glass jars.

Combine curry sauce ingredients in a high-powered blender and blend until smooth.

Bring 3 cups water to a boil, add wild rice, reduce heat to low, and simmer for 40 minutes. Add the edamame and simmer for another 10 minutes, or until the rice is tender and the kernels start to puff open.

Water-sauté the red onion for 3 minutes. Add bok choy stems and mushrooms; cook for another 4–5 minutes until soft. Add bok choy leaves and cook for another 2 minutes or until wilted.

Serve the vegetables over the rice and edamame, topped with curry sauce.

TIP: Frying and sautéing in oil requires large amounts of processed, empty-calorie oil. Water-sauté your vegetables instead.

PER SERVING: CALORIES 294; PROTEIN 15g; CARBOHYDRATES 44g; TOTAL FAT 9g; SATURATED FAT 0.8g; SODIUM 50mg; FIBER 8.7g; BETA-CAROTENE 3,010mcg; VITAMIN C 21mg; CALCIUM 128mg; IRON 3.3mg; FOLATE 223mcg; MAGNESIUM 135mg; ZINC 3.7mg; SELENIUM 21.2mcg

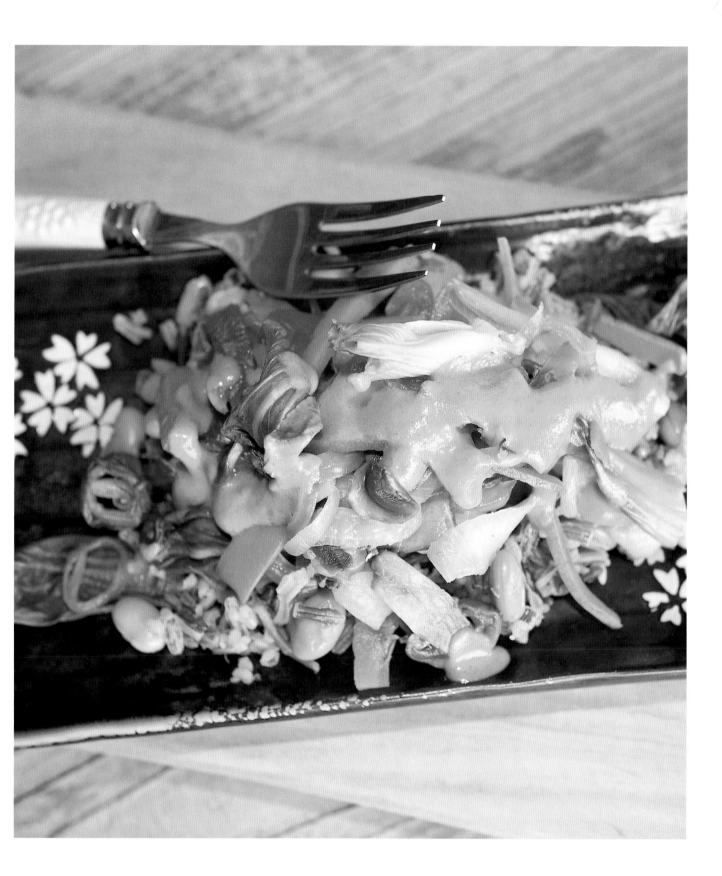

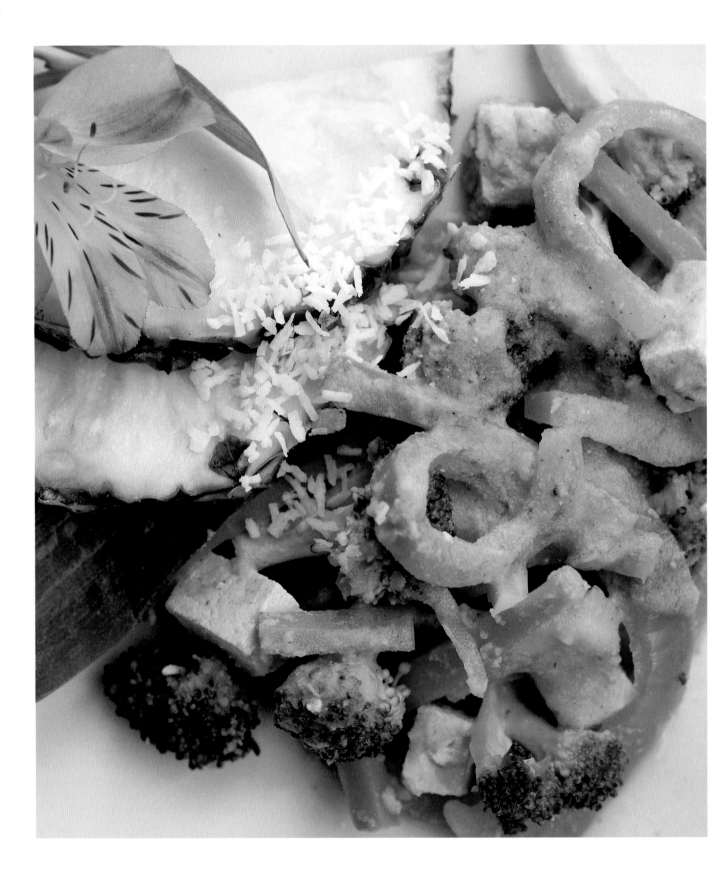

Hawaiian Tofu Stir Fry

Place the tofu in a tofu press or in a colander in the sink with several small plates on top, to remove water from the tofu. When all the water is pressed out, cut the tofu into bite-size squares and place in a storage container.

In a blender, place the shredded coconut, water, pineapple chunks, Bragg Liquid Aminos, scallion, garlic, dried apricots, no-salt seasoning, and vinegar. Blend until smooth. Pour this mixture over the tofu and stir well. Refrigerate for several hours to marinate.

In a wok or large skillet, heat 2 tablespoons vegetable broth over medium high heat. Add the carrot, red onion, and minced ginger. Cook and stir for 7 minutes, adding the remaining vegetable broth if the vegetables begin to stick to the pan. Add the marinated tofu and the broccoli. Stir well. Cover and cook for another 5–10 minutes or until broccoli is tender.

SERVES 4

1 (14-ounce) package firm tofu, well drained

⅓ cup unsweetened, shredded coconut

½ cup water

1 ½ cups pineapple chunks

1 teaspoon Bragg Liquid Aminos or low-sodium soy sauce

1 scallion, sliced (2 tablespoons)

2 cloves garlic, minced

3 unsulfured dried apricots, soaked until soft, drained

½ teaspoon no-salt seasoning such as VegiZest or Mrs. Dash seasoning blend

1 tablespoon passion fruit vinegar or other fruity vinegar

¼ cup low-sodium or no-salt-added vegetable broth

1 carrot, sliced

1 cup sliced red onion

½ teaspoon fresh minced ginger

3 cups broccoli spears

PER SERVING: CALORIES 215; PROTEIN 12g; CARBOHYDRATES 24g; TOTAL FAT 9.5g; SATURATED FAT 4.9g; SODIUM 128mg; FIBER 5.8g; BETA-CAROTENE 1,626mcg; VITAMIN C 96mg; CALCIUM 245mg; IRON 2.6mg; FOLATE 69mcg; MAGNESIUM 37mg; ZINC 0.7mg; SELENIUM 3.7mcg

Very Veggie Burritos or Enchiladas

SERVES 6

1 green bell pepper, seeded and cored

1 medium onion, cut into wedges

3 cloves garlic

1 cup packed, chopped kale

2 cups cooked low-sodium or no-salt-added canned black or red beans, drained

1 ½ cups diced tomatoes

1 cup shredded carrots

1 ½ cups salsa, low-sodium, divided*

2–3 teaspoons chili powder

1 teaspoon cumin

¼ teaspoon red pepper flakes, or to taste

½ avocado

10 whole grain tortillas or 1 head romaine or other leafy lettuce

....

* Dr. Fuhrman's salt-free Tex-Mex Salsa is available at www.drfuhrman.com/shop.

Combine and chop bell pepper, onion, garlic, and kale in a food processor. Remove from food processor and water-sauté mixture in a small amount of water until veggies are very tender.

Add beans, tomatoes, carrots, ½ cup salsa, chili powder, cumin, and red pepper flakes. Stir to combine and simmer until most of the tomato liquid evaporates. Remove from heat.

To make burritos: Blend or mash together remaining 1 cup of salsa with ½ avocado. Spoon beans and veggies onto lettuce leaves or tortillas, top with salsa-avocado mixture and roll tightly.

To make enchiladas: Spoon beans and veggies onto a tortilla, roll, and place in a nonstick or lightly oiled pan. Fill the pan with enchiladas, closely packed together. Spread salsa-avocado mixture thinly across the top of the enchiladas so the tortillas will not crisp up. Bake at 350°F for 20 minutes, or until hot.

Filling may also be used to fill tacos, top a taco salad, or dollop onto crisp vegetable slices such as raw zucchini.

PER SERVING: CALORIES 396; PROTEIN 17g; CARBOHYDRATES 65g; TOTAL FAT 8.5g; SATURATED FAT 1.3g; SODIUM 283mg; FIBER 17.3g; BETA-CAROTENE 3,670mcg; VITAMIN C 55mg; CALCIUM 130mg; IRON 5.8mg; FOLATE 129mcg; MAGNESIUM 68mg; ZINC 1.1mg; SELENIUM 1.5mcg

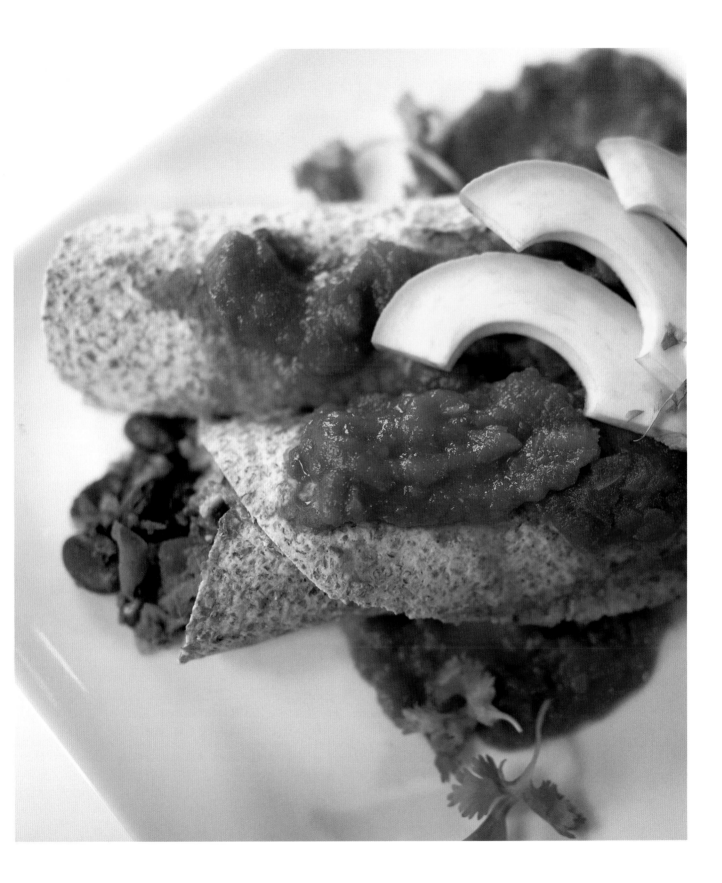

Winter Squash Stuffed with Greens and White Beans

SERVES 4

2 medium acorn or butternut squash, halved and seeded

1 ½ cups cooked or 1 (15-ounce) can no-salt-added or low-sodium white beans, drained, liquid reserved

½ cup chopped onion

2 cloves garlic, chopped

¼ cup no-salt-added tomato sauce

8 cups chopped leafy greens such as kale or Swiss chard

¼ cup pine nuts, toasted

½ teaspoon dried oregano

¼ teaspoon ground black pepper

Preheat oven to 350°F.

Place squash cut side down on a lightly oiled baking pan and bake until tender, about 50–60 minutes.

Meanwhile, heat reserved bean liquid in a large skillet and water-sauté onion and garlic until tender, about 5 minutes. Stir in tomato sauce and greens and cook until greens wilt, about 2 minutes. Stir in white beans, pine nuts, oregano, and black pepper.

Fill each squash half with about 1 cup of the bean mixture. Bake an additional 8–10 minutes at 350° or until filling is heated through.

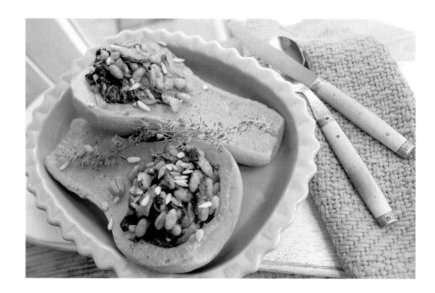

PER SERVING: CALORIES 345; PROTEIN 15g; CARBOHYDRATES 62g; TOTAL FAT 6.8g; SATURATED FAT 0.6g; SODIUM 145mg; FIBER 14.7g; BETA-CAROTENE 3,894mcg; VITAMIN C 44mg; CALCIUM 201mg; IRON 6.8mg; FOLATE 198mcg; MAGNESIUM 201mg; ZINC 2mg; SELENIUM 3.6mcg

Creamy Zoodles

Use a julienne peeler (or a spiral slicer or a regular vegetable peeler) to make "zoodles"—long, thin strips of zucchini that resemble spaghetti noodles.

To make the sauce, combine avocado, basil, lemon juice, garlic, black pepper, Bragg Liquid Aminos, and water in a food processor or high-powered blender and process until smooth and creamy. Add additional water if needed to adjust consistency.

Toss the uncooked (or lightly steamed) zucchini noodles with the sauce. Top with lemon zest.

SERVES 2

3 medium zucchini

1 ripe avocado, peeled and pitted

½ cup fresh basil leaves

1 tablespoon lemon juice

1 clove garlic

⅛ teaspoon ground black pepper

1 teaspoon Bragg Liquid Aminos

1 tablespoon water

1 tablespoon lemon zest

You can substitute bean pasta for the zucchini.

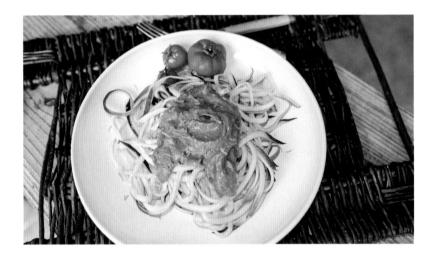

TIP: Thinly sliced or spiralized zucchini is a great replacement for pasta. Zucchini noodles, or "zoodles," are light and tasty and can be served with a variety of healthful toppings.

PER SERVING: CALORIES 172; PROTEIN 6g; CARBOHYDRATES 17g; TOTAL FAT 11.5g; SATURATED FAT 1.7g; SODIUM 141mg; FIBER 8.1g; BETA-CAROTENE 730mcg; VITAMIN C 68mg; CALCIUM 83mg; IRON 1.9mg; FOLATE 140mcg; MAGNESIUM 81mg; ZINC 1.5mg; SELENIUM 1.1mcg

Zucchini Linguini

SERVES 2

2 medium zucchini or yellow squash

3 medium fresh tomatoes, roughly chopped

9 pieces unsalted, unsulfured sun-dried tomatoes, soaked in water for at least 1 hour

2 cloves garlic

4 leaves fresh basil

2 teaspoons balsamic vinegar

Use a julienne peeler (or spiral slicer or regular vegetable peeler) to make long, thin zucchini noodles and arrange on two plates. (If you prefer cooked zucchini, water-sauté it for 2–3 minutes until it is tender but still firm.)

Place fresh tomatoes in a food processor with dried tomatoes and soaking water, garlic, basil, and vinegar. Pulse until you reach desired consistency. Spoon the sauce over the zucchini.

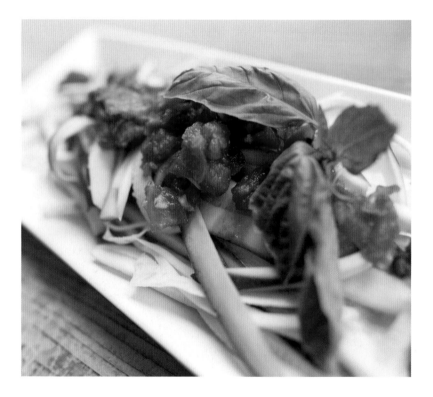

PER SERVING: CALORIES 113; PROTEIN 6g; CARBOHYDRATES 23g; TOTAL FAT 1.4g; SATURATED FAT 0.3g; SODIUM 43mg; FIBER 6g; BETA-CAROTENE 1,229mcg; VITAMIN C 67mg; CALCIUM 75mg; IRON 2.6mg; FOLATE 85mcg; MAGNESIUM 85mg; ZINC 1.3mg; SELENIUM 0.8mcg

QUICK WHOLE GRAIN MAIN DISHES

Intact whole grains are the best choice for grain products.

Intact grains still retain the shape and appearance of the way they were grown and harvested. They have not been ground into flour. Because they are not ground and contain the full fibrous shell, intact grains are digested slowly and have a more favorable glycemic index.

Creamy Barley Risotto with Tomatoes and Peas

SERVES 4

1 medium onion, chopped

1 clove garlic, minced

1 ½ cups whole grain barley

½ teaspoon dried basil

½ teaspoon dried oregano

1 ½ cups chopped tomatoes

1 ½ cups unsweetened, unflavored soy, hemp, or almond milk

2 cups water

¼ cup unfortified nutritional yeast

½ tablespoon reduced-sodium miso, mixed with 1 tablespoon water

1 cup thawed frozen peas

Hulled and hull-less barley are two different varieties of barley; both are considered whole grains. Quicker-cooking pearl barley has been refined and is not a whole grain.

Heat 2–3 tablespoons water in a medium-size pot and water-sauté onion until tender. Add garlic and cook another minute. Add remaining ingredients. Stir well, bring to a boil, reduce heat, partially cover, and simmer until barley is tender and liquid is absorbed, stirring occasionally, about 75 minutes.

The mixture should be creamy but not soupy, and the barley will be chewy, not mushy.

PER SERVING: CALORIES 344; PROTEIN 16g; CARBOHYDRATES 64g; TOTAL FAT 3.4g; SATURATED FAT 0.5g; SODIUM 206mg; FIBER 16.6g; BETA-CAROTENE 726mcg; VITAMIN C 18mg; CALCIUM 254mg; IRON 4.2mg; FOLATE 49mcg; MAGNESIUM 132mg; ZINC 4.1mg; SELENIUM 27.1mcg

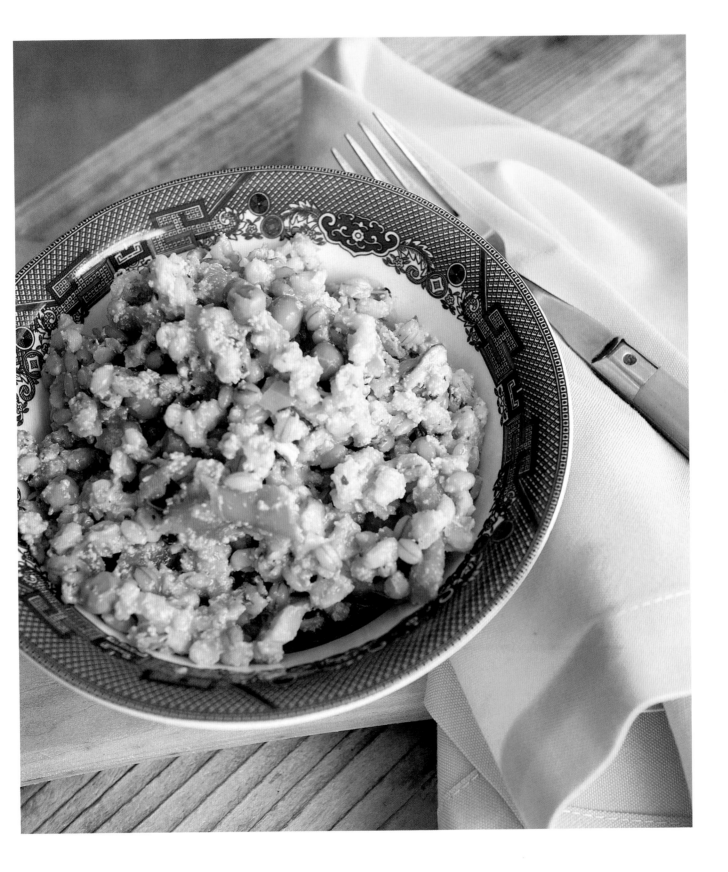

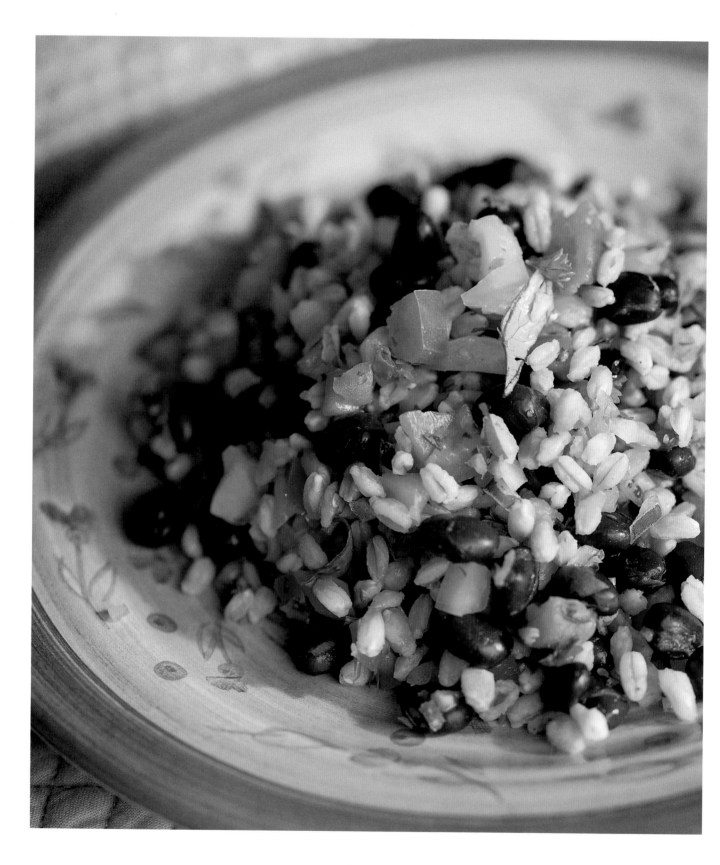

Farro with Black Beans and Fresh Herbs

Look for whole grain or semi-pearled farro. Pearled farro cooks faster, but the nutritious germ and bran have been removed.

Cook farro according to package instructions. Place in a large bowl and mix in remaining ingredients.

SERVES 4

1 cup farro (whole grain or semi-pearled)

1 small red bell pepper, finely diced

1 small yellow or orange pepper, finely diced

½ red onion, finely diced

2 tablespoons chopped parsley

2 tablespoons chopped cilantro

1 small lemon, juiced

1 ½ cups cooked or 1 (15-ounce) can low-sodium or no-salt-added black beans, drained

½ teaspoon garlic powder

Black pepper, to taste

¼ teaspoon cumin (optional)

PER SERVING: CALORIES 313; PROTEIN 13g; CARBOHYDRATES 59g; TOTAL FAT 1.9g; SATURATED FAT 0.1g; SODIUM 6mg; FIBER 13.8g; BETA-CAROTENE 445mcg; VITAMIN C 75mg; CALCIUM 70mg; IRON 4.3mg; FOLATE 83mcg; MAGNESIUM 43mg; ZINC 0.7mg; SELENIUM 1.1mcg

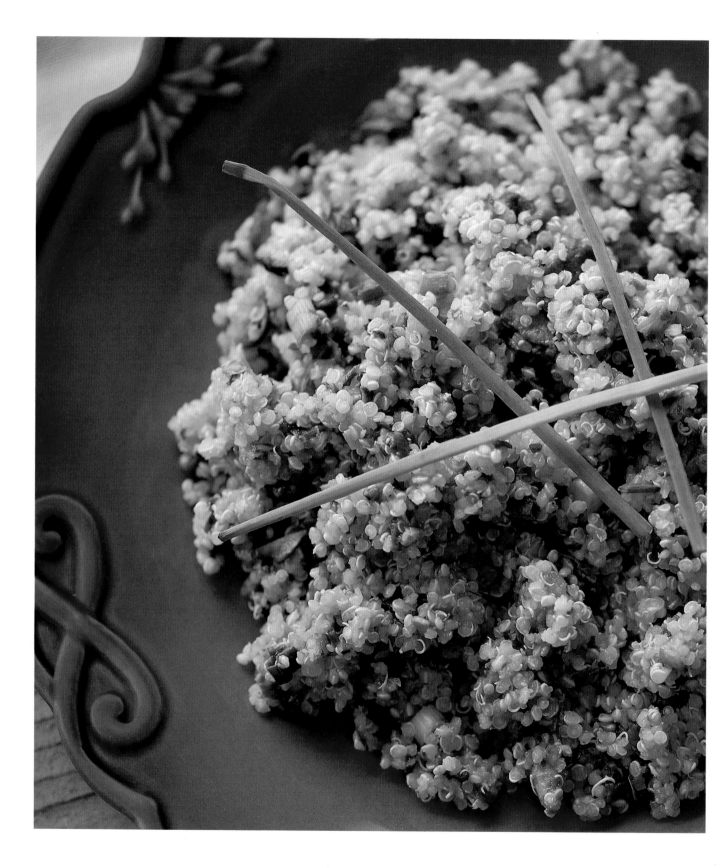

Lemony Mushroom Quinoa

Rinse quinoa in cold water, and drain. Combine quinoa and vegetable stock, and cook covered about 15 minutes, on medium heat, or until quinoa is done.

While quinoa is cooking, place mushrooms in a sauté pan over medium heat. When mushrooms begin to give off juice, add garlic and continue to cook until mushrooms are cooked to your liking. Place quinoa, mushrooms, and remaining ingredients in a large bowl and gently combine. Serve at room temperature.

SERVES 4

1 cup quinoa

2 cups low-sodium or no-salt-added vegetable stock

1 pound fresh mushrooms, chopped

2 cloves fresh garlic, finely chopped

4 green onions, white and light green parts, finely sliced

¼ cup chopped fresh parsley

2 tablespoons chopped fresh chives

1 fresh lemon, juiced and zested

¼ cup white balsamic vinegar

1 teaspoon freshly ground black pepper

PER SERVING: CALORIES 225; PROTEIN 12g; CARBOHYDRATES 38g; TOTAL FAT 3.8g; SATURATED FAT 0.6g; SODIUM 52mg; FIBER 4.7g; BETA-CAROTENE 525mcg; VITAMIN C 13mg; CALCIUM 52mg; IRON 3.3mg; FOLATE 110mcg; MAGNESIUM 104mg; ZINC 2.1mg; SELENIUM 14.5mcg

Wild Rice with Apricots and Sesame Seeds

SERVES 6

2 cups wild rice

¼ teaspoon ground cumin

½ teaspoon coriander

½ teaspoon cinnamon

1 cup unsulfured dried apricots, coarsely chopped

3 cups water

¼ cup unhulled sesame seeds

Cook rice, spices, and dried apricots with water on low heat for 35 minutes. Add sesame seeds and simmer for 10 more minutes or until rice is cooked.

PER SERVING: CALORIES 278; PROTEIN 10g; CARBOHYDRATES 55g; TOTAL FAT 3.7g; SATURATED FAT 0.5g; SODIUM 13mg; FIBER 5.8g; BETA-CAROTENE 476mcg; CALCIUM 89mg; IRON 2.6mg; FOLATE 59mcg; MAGNESIUM 125mg; ZINC 3.8mg; SELENIUM 4.1mcg

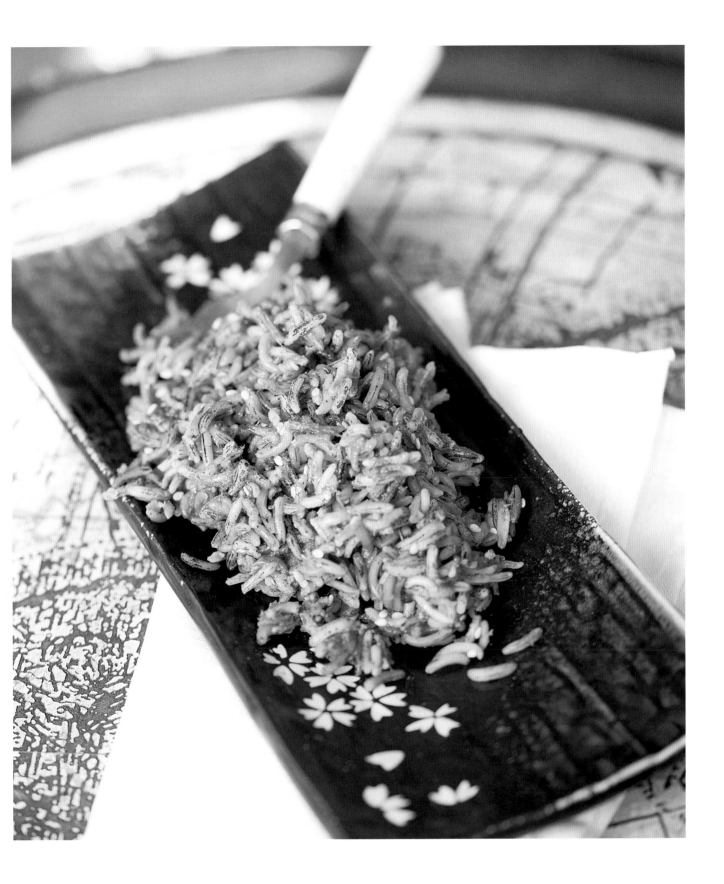

NON-VEGAN MAIN DISHES

The Nutritarian diet is not an all-or-nothing eating plan. You can adjust it to your needs and personal preferences. The goal is to stay within certain boundaries so you still reap the dramatic health and lifespan benefits.

If you want to use meat or dairy products in your diet, just don't eat a large portion at any meal. Instead, use them in small amounts as a condiment or flavoring. The goal is to keep animal product intake to levels below 5 percent of total calories, or less than 8–10 ounces per week. Be sure to choose clean, wild-caught fish and certified organic meat or poultry.

Complete veganism scares some people away from trying a vegan diet. The good news is that you can get the health benefits of a vegan diet without having to be completely vegan. The recipes in this section show how a little bit of scallops, chicken, turkey, or wild meat can be added to many of the dishes in this book, in small amounts, to enhance flavor. You can even make a mostly veggie burger that tastes like you are eating meat—the trick is to chop the meat finely or shred it into small pieces so that the flavor is dispersed in every mouthful. It is amazing that adding only 1 ounce of animal product per serving can please meat lovers and still enable them to comply with a high-vegetable, Nutritarian diet.

Chicken-Seasoned Quinoa

SERVES 6

1 (6-ounce) chicken breast

3 cups low-sodium or no-salt-added vegetable broth

1 onion, chopped

10 large shiitake or other mushrooms, coarsely chopped

1 ½ cups quinoa, rinsed in a fine mesh strainer

1 red bell pepper, cut into thin strips

½ cup thawed frozen peas

1 cup cooked chickpeas

1 cup cherry or grape tomatoes, halved

2 cups spinach, chopped

¼ cup fresh basil, chopped

2 tablespoons lemon juice

Black pepper, to taste

Place chicken breast in a saucepan and add 2 tablespoons low-sodium vegetable broth to partially cover. Bring to a boil, reduce heat, cover, and simmer 15–20 minutes or until cooked through. Drain (setting aside the broth) and cool, then shred into pieces.

Heat 2 tablespoons broth in a large skillet; add onion and mushrooms and sauté until soft. Add the quinoa, red pepper, and vegetable broth. Bring to a boil, reduce heat, and cook covered for 15 minutes. Stir in peas and continue cooking until quinoa is tender and all liquid is absorbed.

Stir in shredded chicken, chickpeas, tomatoes, spinach, basil, and lemon juice. Season with black pepper.

Serve warm or at room temperature.

PER SERVING: CALORIES 301; PROTEIN 19g; CARBOHYDRATES 47g; TOTAL FAT 4.5g; SATURATED FAT 0.7g; CHOLESTEROL 21.8mg; SODIUM 114mg; FIBER 7.5g; BETA-CAROTENE 1,127mcg; VITAMIN C 38mg; CALCIUM 76mg; IRON 4.0mg; FOLATE 176mcg; MAGNESIUM 127mg; ZINC 2.7mg; SELENIUM 15.4mcg

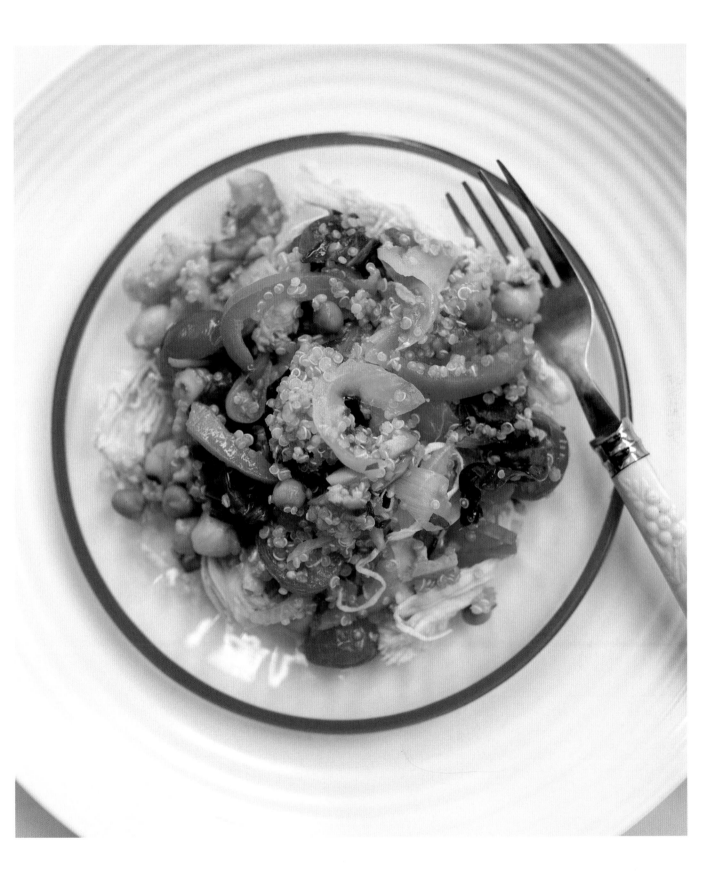

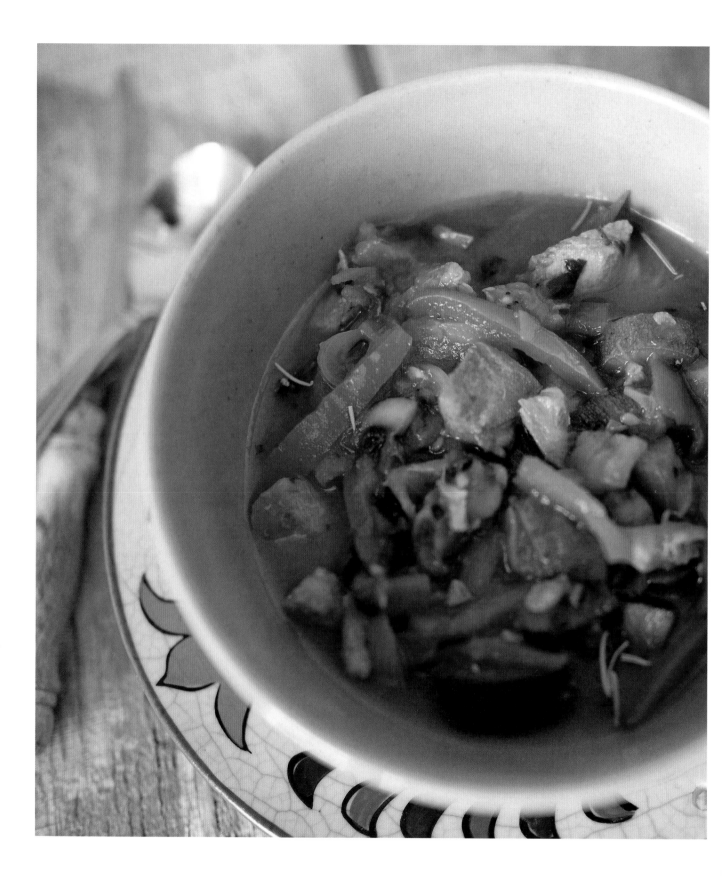

Quick Fish and White Bean Stew

Heat ⅛ cup water on medium heat in a large pan. Add the bell peppers and onions and cook for 3 minutes; add the zucchini and mushrooms and continue cooking for another 6–8 minutes or until tender, adding more water if necessary to keep vegetables from sticking.

Add the tomatoes, beans, garlic, Herbes de Provence, and black pepper and simmer on low heat for 4 minutes. Add the fish to the stew and mix in gently. Cover and simmer on low heat for 8–10 minutes, stirring occasionally.

Before serving, stir in lemon juice.

SERVES 4

2 red bell peppers, sliced

2 medium onions, sliced

2 medium zucchini, cut into 1-inch pieces

2 cups sliced mushrooms

6 medium tomatoes, chopped

1 ½ cups cooked or 1 (15-ounce) can no-salt-added or low-sodium white beans, drained

2 cloves garlic, finely chopped

1 teaspoon Herbes de Provence

¼ teaspoon black pepper

⅓ pound firm fish fillets (such as halibut, bass, salmon), cut into 1-inch pieces

1 tablespoon fresh lemon juice

PER SERVING: CALORIES 235; PROTEIN 19g; CARBOHYDRATES 35g; TOTAL FAT 3.2g; SATURATED FAT 0.7g; CHOLESTEROL 17mg; SODIUM 30mg; FIBER 13g; BETA-CAROTENE 1,798mcg; VITAMIN C 110mg; CALCIUM 119mg; IRON 3.9mg; FOLATE 132mcg; MAGNESIUM 93mg; ZINC 1.9mg; SELENIUM 18.5mcg

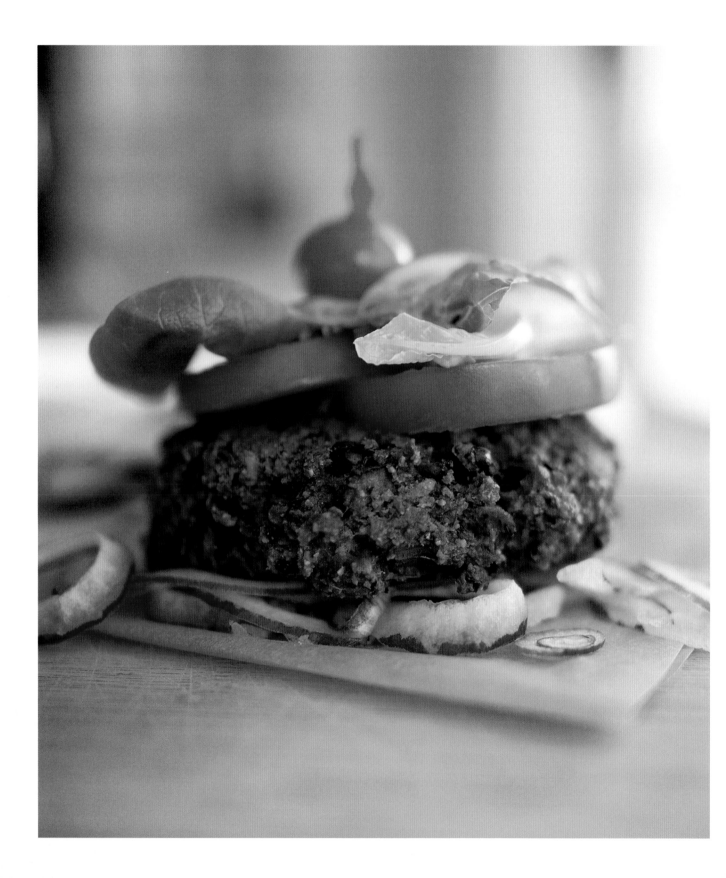

Black Bean, Beef, and Mushroom Burgers

Preheat oven to 300°F.

Heat 1–2 tablespoons water in a small pan and water-sauté mushrooms until tender and moisture has evaporated, about 5 minutes. Set aside.

Grind oats and pumpkin seeds in a food processor. Add 1 cup of the beans, plus the basil, oregano, and black pepper and process until blended.

Spoon mixture into a mixing bowl and stir in sautéed mushrooms, remaining whole beans, and ground beef. Form into seven medium-size patties. Add additional oats if needed to help form burgers.

Place patties on a baking sheet lined with parchment paper or lightly wiped with olive oil. Bake 40 minutes, turning once after 20 minutes.

Serve on a small 100 percent whole grain roll or pita with sliced red onion, sliced tomato, lettuce, and a low-sodium, no-corn-syrup ketchup.

SERVES 7

2 cups chopped mushrooms

½ cup old-fashioned rolled oats

¼ cup raw pumpkin seeds

1 ½ cups cooked or 1 (15-ounce) can low-sodium or no-salt-added black beans, drained and divided

1 teaspoon dry basil

½ teaspoon oregano

⅛ teaspoon black pepper

6 ounces (about 1 cup) organic ground beef*

To make burgers without ground beef, blend an additional 1 ½ cups beans with the oat and pumpkin seed mixture.

Dr. Fuhrman's Nutritarian Ketchup is available at www.drfuhrman.com/shop.

PER SERVING: CALORIES 145; PROTEIN 11g; CARBOHYDRATES 14g; TOTAL FAT 5.4g; SATURATED FAT 1.5g; CHOLESTEROL 15.8mg; SODIUM 18mg; FIBER 4.5g; BETA-CAROTENE 3,608mcg; VITAMIN C 1mg; CALCIUM 31mg; IRON 3.8mg; FOLATE 65mcg; MAGNESIUM 65mg; ZINC 2.1mg; SELENIUM 6.9mcg

Quick Turkey and Bean Burgers

SERVES 6

½ medium green bell pepper, cut into large pieces

½ medium onion

2 cloves garlic

1 ½ cups cooked or 1 (15-ounce) can no-salt-added or low-sodium black beans, drained

6 ounces organic ground turkey

2 teaspoons chili powder

2 teaspoons cumin

Preheat oven to 350°F.

Place the bell pepper, onion, and garlic in a food processor and pulse until finely chopped. Add the black beans and pulse to combine and chop up the beans. Place mixture in a medium bowl and stir in the ground turkey, chili powder, and cumin.

Divide the mixture into six patties. Place on a baking sheet lined with parchment paper or lightly wiped with oil. Bake 40 minutes, turning after 20 minutes.

Serve on a small 100 percent whole grain roll or pita with sliced red onion, sliced tomato, and lettuce.

PER SERVING: CALORIES 112; PROTEIN 13g; CARBOHYDRATES 13g; TOTAL FAT 1.3g; SATURATED FAT 0.3g; CHOLESTEROL 20.8mg; SODIUM 37mg; FIBER 4.5g; BETA-CAROTENE 169mcg; VITAMIN C 12mg; CALCIUM 28mg; IRON 1.9mg; FOLATE 71mcg; MAGNESIUM 47mg; ZINC 1.3mg; SELENIUM 9.3mcg

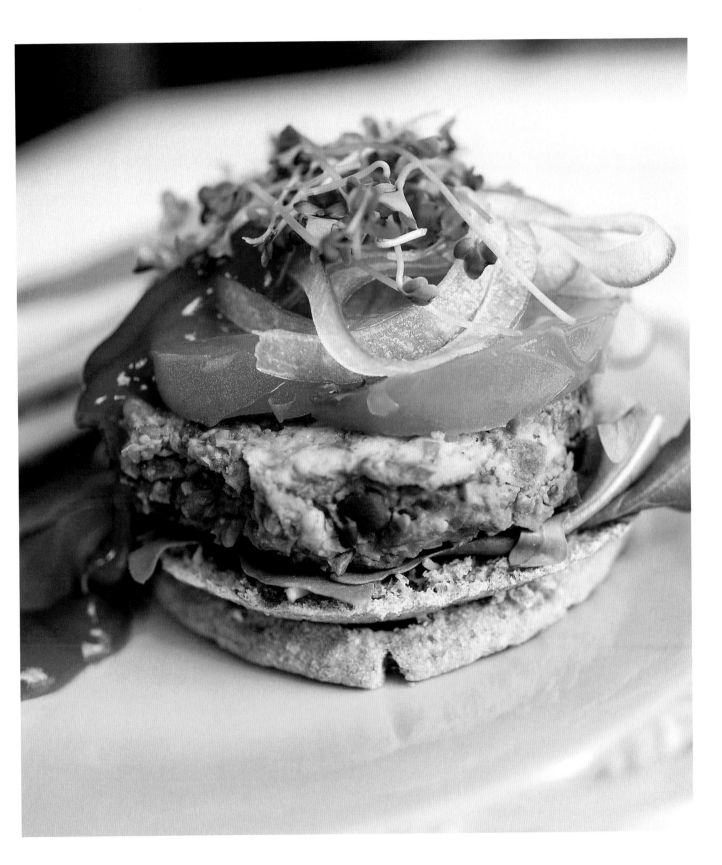

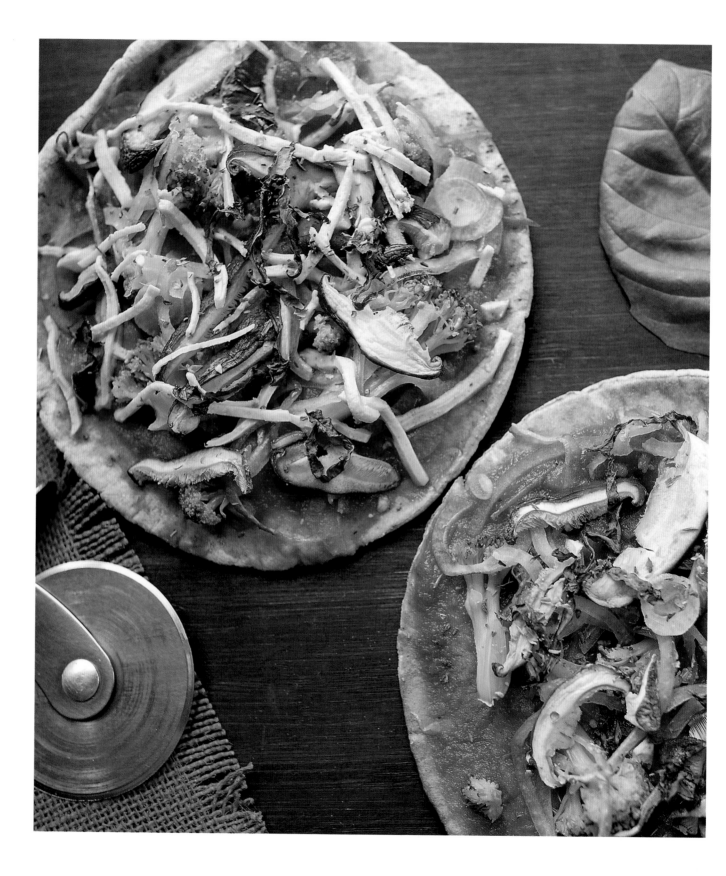

Easy Vegetable Pizza

Preheat oven to 200°F.

Place tortillas or pitas on two baking sheets and warm for 10 minutes. Remove from oven and spoon on the pasta sauce. Sprinkle evenly with mushrooms, onions, and broccoli. Add a light sprinkle of cheese. Bake 30 minutes.

SERVES 4

4 large (100% whole grain) tortillas or pitas

2 cups no-salt-added or low-sodium tomato-based pasta sauce

½ cup chopped shiitake mushrooms

½ cup chopped red onions

10 ounces frozen broccoli florets, thawed and finely chopped

4 tablespoons shredded mozzarella cheese*

You can use a nondairy mozzarella or omit the cheese.

PER SERVING: CALORIES 250; PROTEIN 12g; CARBOHYDRATES 40g; TOTAL FAT 6.2g; SATURATED FAT 1g; CHOLESTEROL 1.1mg; SODIUM 219mg; FIBER 9.7g; BETA-CAROTENE 752mcg; VITAMIN C 50mg; CALCIUM 150mg; IRON 4mg; FOLATE 70mcg; MAGNESIUM 39mg; ZINC 1.1mg; SELENIUM 7.9mcg

Stuffed Peppers with Mushrooms, Greens, and Ground Turkey

12 ounces lean ground turkey

1 onion, chopped

½ cup whole garlic cloves, chopped

2 cups sliced mushrooms

4 cups chopped greens, such as kale or collards

2 cups water

1 cup wild rice

1 cup raw pumpkin seeds

1 teaspoon hot sauce, if desired

6 whole green or red bell peppers, halved, seeds removed

Preheat oven to 250°F.

Cook turkey in a skillet lightly coated with cooking spray or olive oil. Stir in chopped onion, garlic, mushrooms, and greens. Allow to steam slightly. Add 2 cups water and then stir in the rice. Cook covered 30 minutes or until rice is tender.

Add pumpkin seeds and hot sauce, if desired.

Place peppers hollow side up in a baking dish and stuff with turkey mixture. Bake, covered, for 1 hour or until peppers are tender.

PER SERVING: CALORIES 325; PROTEIN 24g; CARBOHYDRATES 22g; TOTAL FAT 17.5g; SATURATED FAT 3.7g; CHOLESTEROL 55.9mg; SODIUM 133mg; FIBER 4.8g; BETA-CAROTENE 815mcg; VITAMIN C 106mg; CALCIUM 80mg; IRON 3.9mg; FOLATE 58mcg; MAGNESIUM 184mg; ZINC 4.4mg; SELENIUM 27.4mcg

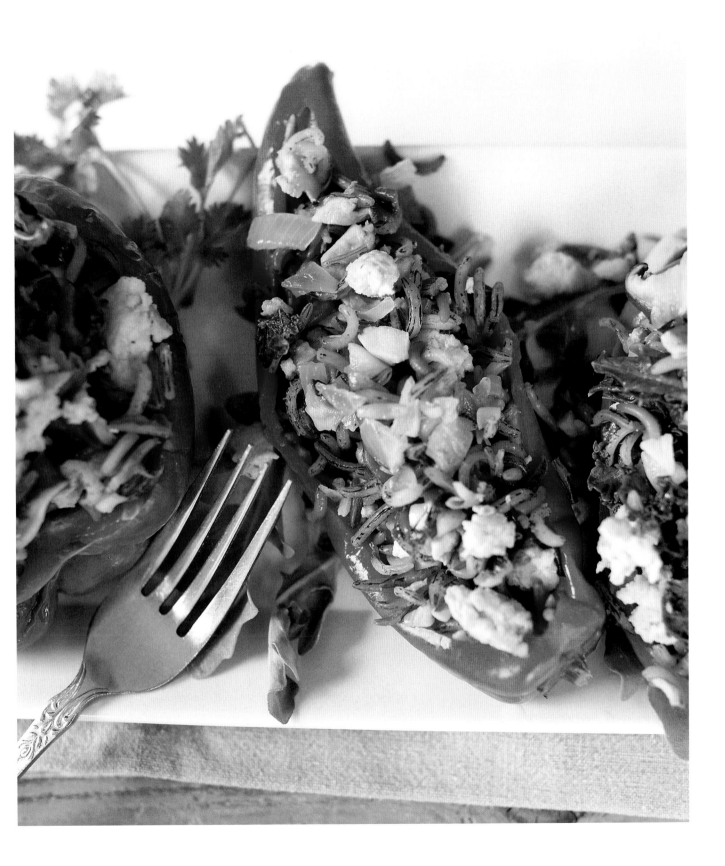

BURGERS, PIZZAS, AND WRAPS

*Eat for health . . . your ideal weight and many
other wondrous things will follow!*

Fast-food meals of the Standard American Diet (SAD) are off the charts when it comes to calories, sodium, and fat, and they offer paltry amounts of fiber, vitamins, and minerals. A typical fast-food meal consisting of a burger (two all-beef patties, "special" sauce, and a sesame seed bun), medium fries, and a 32-ounce soda weighs in at 1,480 calories, 1,490 grams sodium, and 48 grams fat. And that's the worst type of fat to eat, too.

Make your own better-for-you burgers, pizzas, and wraps. Bean burgers, veggie pizzas, and vegetable-stuffed wraps and pitas will leave you feeling so much better, both physically and mentally.

Always choose 100 percent whole grain breads and wraps. Look for bread products that are made from intact sprouted grains or coarsely ground grain. Manna Organics bread and Food for Life's Ezekiel bread are examples of national brands whose grains are more intact and therefore are good choices. They are available in the frozen section of many supermarkets and health food stores.

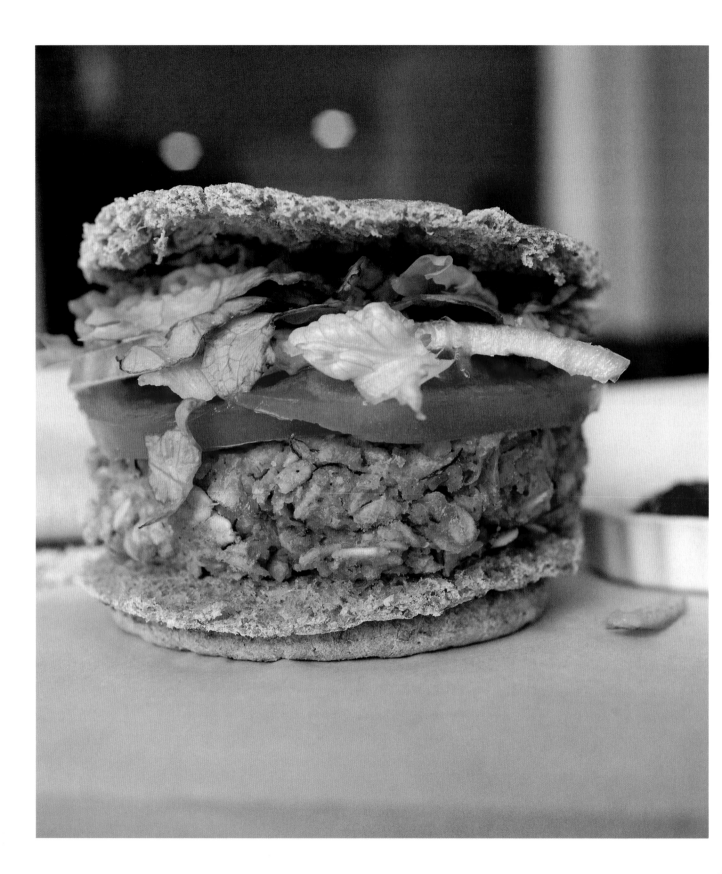

Chickpea Burgers

Preheat oven to 350°F.

Place chickpeas in a bowl and mash with a fork. Add remaining ingredients and mix well. Form into six patties.

Place on a baking sheet lined with parchment paper or lightly wiped with oil. Bake 15 minutes, turn, and bake an additional 10 minutes.

Serve on 100% whole grain buns or pitas if desired, topped with tomato, red onion slices, and lettuce.

SERVES 6

1 ½ cups cooked or 1 (15-ounce) can low-sodium or no-salt-added chickpeas (garbanzo beans), drained

¼ cup finely diced red onion

½ cup grated zucchini

2 tablespoons red wine vinegar

2 tablespoons low-sodium ketchup*

2 tablespoons low-sodium, natural peanut butter

1 teaspoon cumin

1 teaspoon garlic powder

¼ teaspoon black pepper

1 cup old-fashioned oats

....

* Dr. Fuhrman's Nutritarian Ketchup is available at www.drfuhrman.com/shop.

TIP: Achieve permanent weight control and superior health by eating more nutrient-rich foods and fewer high-calorie, low-nutrient foods. The more high-nutrient foods you consume, the fewer low-nutrient foods you desire.

PER SERVING: CALORIES 162; PROTEIN 7g; CARBOHYDRATES 24g; TOTAL FAT 4.9g; SATURATED FAT 0.7g; SODIUM 17mg; FIBER 5.1g; BETA-CAROTENE 50mcg; VITAMIN C 4mg; CALCIUM 31mg; IRON 5mg; FOLATE 80mcg; MAGNESIUM 34mg; ZINC 0.9mg; SELENIUM 2.1mcg

Tofu Pizza Bites

SERVES 2

1 (12-ounce) package extra firm tofu

1 cup low-sodium or no-salt-added tomato-based pasta sauce*

2 tablespoons tomato paste*

1 teaspoon garlic powder

1 teaspoon onion powder

---

* Choose tomato products packaged in BPA-free materials such as cartons or glass.

Baked tofu substitutes for the crust in this easy, kid-friendly pizza.

Cut tofu into thin slices and place on a wire rack.

Mix the tomato sauce and tomato paste with the spices and spread over the tofu. Bake in a 325°F oven for 30 minutes or until tofu is hardened and yellowed on the outside.

PER SERVING: CALORIES 181; PROTEIN 15g; CARBOHYDRATES 19g; TOTAL FAT 5.2g; SATURATED FAT 0.8g; CHOLESTEROL 2.6mg; SODIUM 157mg; FIBER 3.5g; BETA-CAROTENE 645mcg; VITAMIN C 6mg; CALCIUM 99mg; IRON 3.6mg; FOLATE 20mcg; MAGNESIUM 78mg; ZINC 1.5mg; SELENIUM 2.8mcg

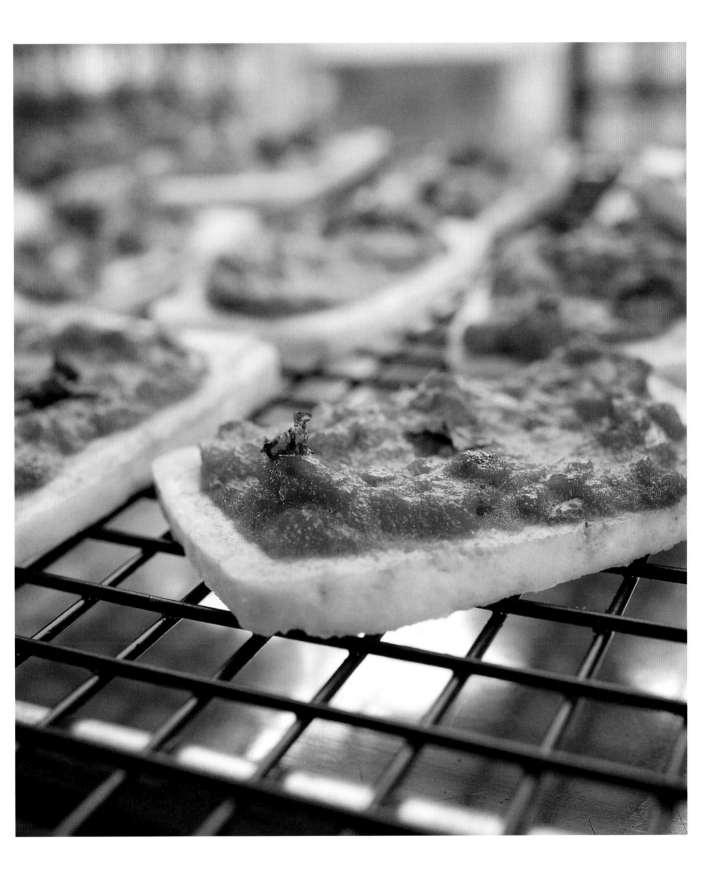

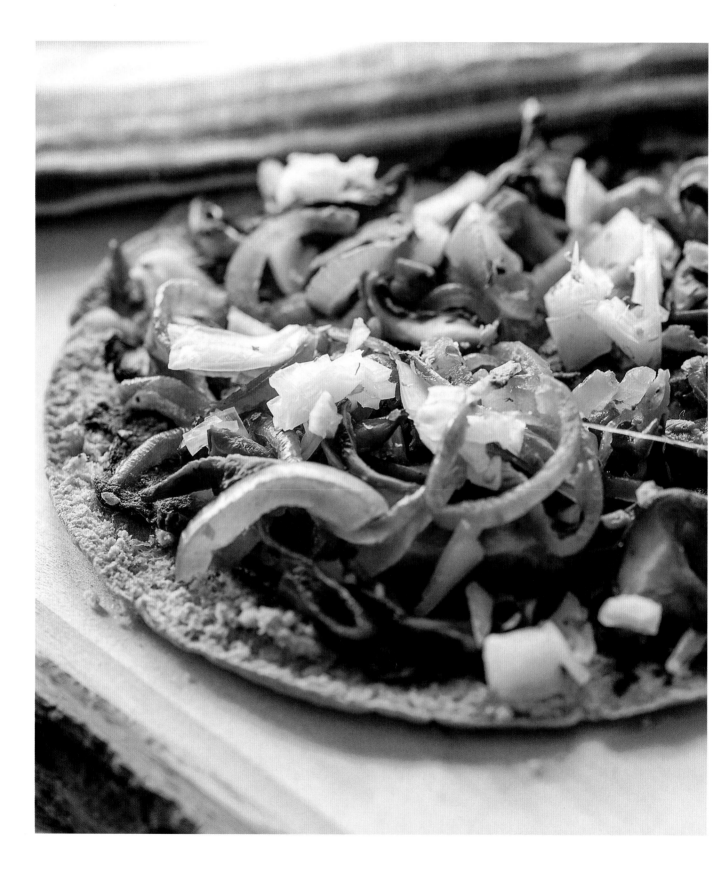

Mushroom, Onion, and Pesto Pizza

To make the pesto, add the garlic, walnuts, vinegar, water, Italian seasoning, and unfortified nutritional yeast to a food processor or blender and blend at high speed. Turn to low speed and add the arugula and spinach. Blend to a chunky consistency. Set aside.

Preheat oven to 350°F.

Heat 2–3 tablespoons water in a large pan and water-sauté red onion 1–2 minutes; add mushrooms and continue to cook until onions are tender and liquid from mushrooms has cooked off.

Bake tortillas or pitas directly on oven rack for 5–7 minutes or until just crisp.

Spread a thin layer of pesto sauce on each tortilla or pita and top with the sautéed onions and mushrooms. Top with chopped fresh tomato.

Bake an additional 3–5 minutes or until toppings are warm, checking occasionally to avoid browning of vegetables.

SERVES 4

For the pesto

2 cloves garlic

½ cup walnuts

¼ cup balsamic vinegar

½ cup water

½ tablespoon no-salt Italian seasoning, adjusted to taste

½ tablespoon unfortified nutritional yeast

2 cups arugula

2 cups spinach

For the pizza

1 large onion, sliced

10 ounces mushrooms, sliced

4 (100% whole grain) tortillas or pitas

1 medium tomato, chopped

PER SERVING: CALORIES 297; PROTEIN 12g; CARBOHYDRATES 38g; TOTAL FAT 12.2g; SATURATED FAT 1.4g; SODIUM 169mg; FIBER 8.4g; BETA-CAROTENE 1,126mcg; VITAMIN C 15mg; CALCIUM 109mg; IRON 3.8mg; FOLATE 79mcg; MAGNESIUM 56mg; ZINC 1.2mg; SELENIUM 7.8mcg

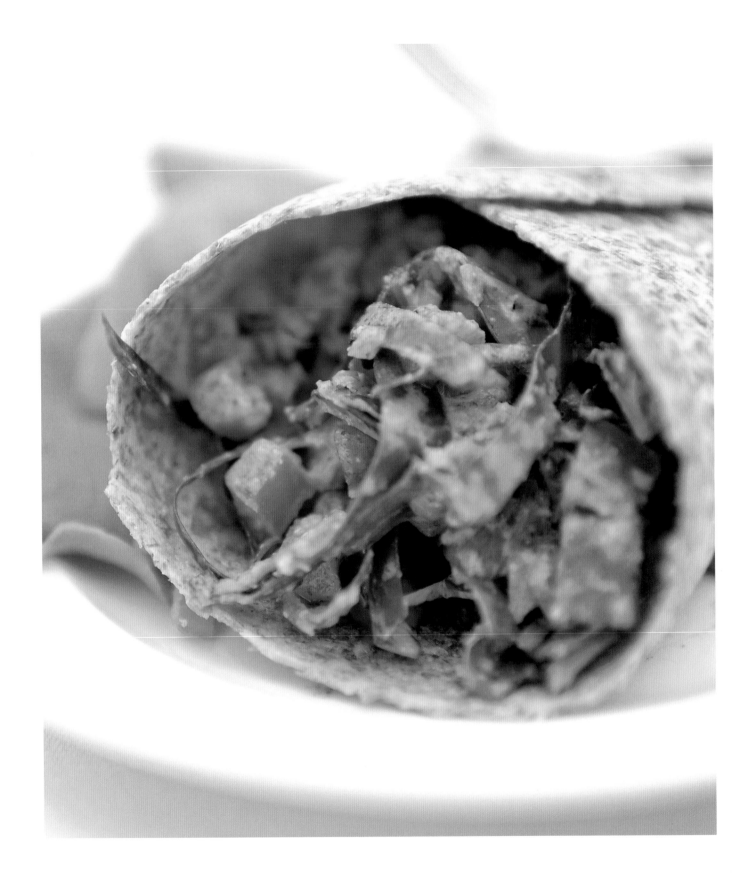

Mediterranean Collard Green Wraps

In a bowl, mix together collard greens, salsa, almond butter, cilantro, cumin, and chili powder. Serve stuffed into a whole grain pita or wrap.

SERVES 2

2 cups very finely shredded collard greens

¼ cup low-sodium salsa*

¼ cup raw almond butter

¼ cup fresh cilantro, minced

1 teaspoon ground cumin

1 teaspoon chili powder

2 (100% whole grain) wraps or pitas

* Dr. Fuhrman's salt-free Tex-Mex Salsa is available at www.drfuhrman.com/shop.

PER SERVING: CALORIES 385; PROTEIN 14g; CARBOHYDRATES 45g; TOTAL FAT 19.6g; SATURATED FAT 1.6g; SODIUM 376mg; FIBER 10.2g; BETA-CAROTENE 1,774mcg; VITAMIN C 16mg; CALCIUM 188mg; IRON 4.1mg; FOLATE 104mcg; MAGNESIUM 143mg; ZINC 2.2mg; SELENIUM 29.7mcg

Speedy Vegetable Wraps

SERVES 2

2 (100% whole grain) flour tortillas

1 tablespoon fat-free, low-sodium dressing*

2 cups broccoli slaw mix**

1 tablespoon diced red onion

1 large tomato, diced

½ avocado, sliced

....

Look for dressings that have no refined oil and contain less than 150 mg sodium per 2 tablespoons. Some choices include Dr. Fuhrman's bottled dressings (available online at www.drfuhrman.com), Annie's Naturals Fat Free Raspberry Balsamic Vinaigrette, and Maple Grove Farms Fat Free Balsamic Vinaigrette.

**You can buy prepackaged broccoli slaw in the produce section of many markets. You can also use cole slaw mix, shredded cabbage, or shredded broccoli.*

Spread tortillas with dressing. Add broccoli slaw mix, onion, tomato, and avocado to tortillas and roll up.

You can also make these with 100% whole grain pita bread.

PER SERVING: CALORIES 266; PROTEIN 13g; CARBOHYDRATES 35g; TOTAL FAT 9.2g; SATURATED FAT 1.5g; CHOLESTEROL 2.4mg; SODIUM 295mg; FIBER 8.7g; BETA-CAROTENE 2,938mcg; VITAMIN C 75mg; CALCIUM 205mg; IRON 3mg; FOLATE 65mcg; MAGNESIUM 33mg; ZINC 1mg; SELENIUM 4.1mcg

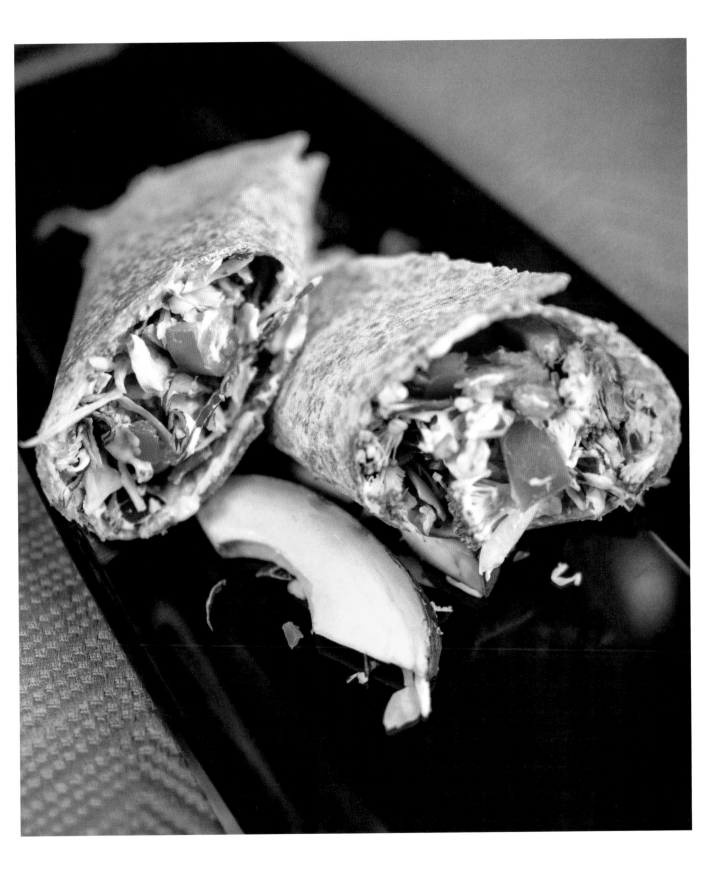

Sautéed Kale and Chickpea Pitas

SERVES 4

½ to 1 cup low-sodium vegetable broth

3 cloves garlic, minced

1 bunch kale, tough stems removed, chopped

¼ teaspoon hot pepper flakes

1 ½ cups cooked or 1 (15-ounce) can low-sodium or no-salt-added chickpeas, drained

¼ cup low-sodium, no-oil dressing, or low-sodium, no-corn-syrup ketchup or homemade healthy mayo*

4 (100% whole grain) pitas or 4 slices of 100% whole grain bread such as Ezekiel

1 small red onion, very thinly sliced

....

To make homemade healthy mayo, blend 1 cup raw cashews, ¼ cup sunflower seeds, 3 tablespoons apple cider vinegar, 2 tablespoons lemon juice, 2 tablespoons water, 2 pitted dates, and 1 clove garlic in a high-powered blender. Dr. Fuhrman's Nutritarian Ketchup, Nuttynaise, and salad dressings are also super-healthy options for these sandwiches. They are available at www.drfuhrman.com/shop.

Heat ½ cup vegetable broth in a large sauté pan, add garlic, and simmer for 1 minute; then add kale and hot pepper flakes. Cover and simmer over low heat for 5 minutes.

Add chickpeas and additional vegetable broth as needed, and simmer for an additional 15 minutes. Mash some of the chickpeas with a fork or the back of a spoon.

Spread some of the dressing, ketchup, or homemade mayo on pitas or, for an open-face sandwich, on a slice of 100% whole grain bread.

Add kale and chickpeas and top with sliced red onion.

PER SERVING: CALORIES 235; PROTEIN 10g; CARBOHYDRATES 46g; TOTAL FAT 2.4g; SATURATED FAT 0.2g; SODIUM 151mg; FIBER 8.8g; BETA-CAROTENE 4,638mcg; VITAMIN C 48mg; CALCIUM 92mg; IRON 3.7mg; FOLATE 121mcg; MAGNESIUM 47mg; ZINC 1.2mg; SELENIUM 3.1mcg

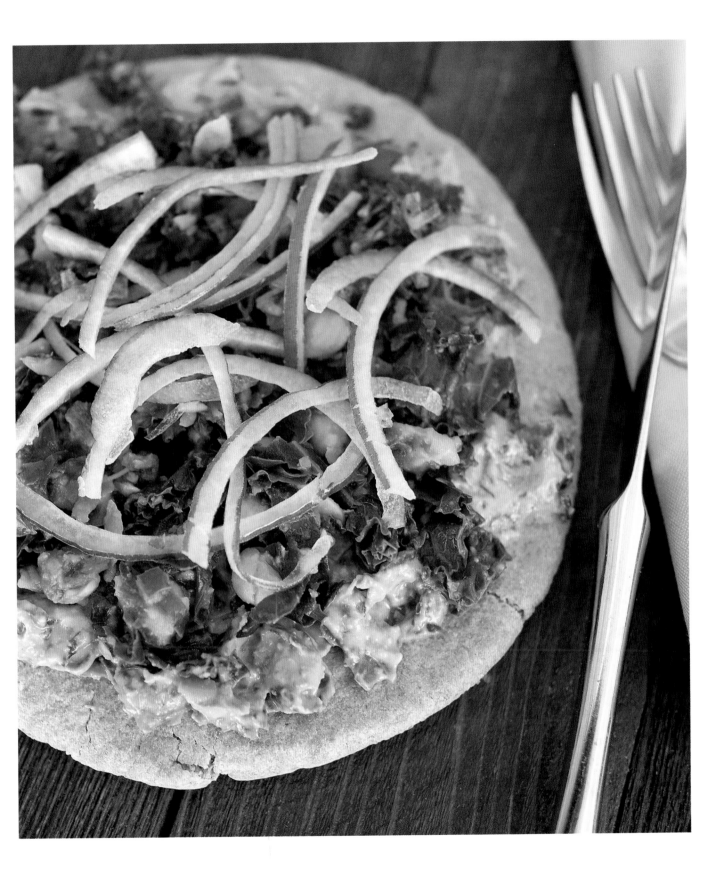

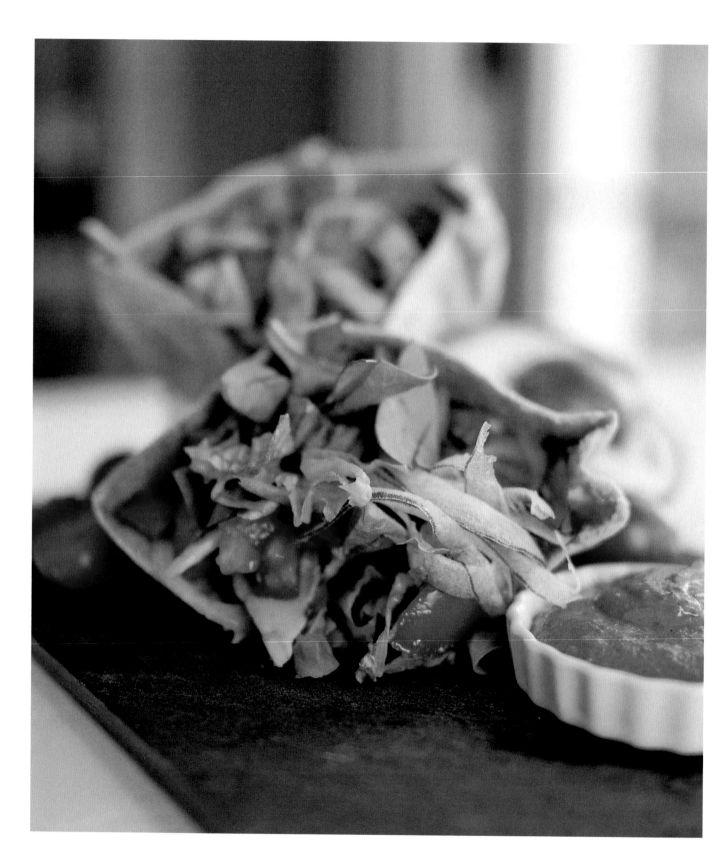

Tomato Almond Pocket Pitas

Combine almonds, pasta sauce, and a splash of vinegar to make a flavorful sandwich spread.

Lightly toast the pitas. Use a fork to mash the almond butter with the pasta sauce, vinegar, and chili powder until it has a smooth consistency. If using raw almonds, blend ingredients together in a high-powered blender.

Cut pitas in half to form a pocket. Stuff with almond butter mixture, avocado, tomato, lettuce, spinach, and red onion.

SERVES 4

4 (100% whole grain) pitas

¼ cup raw almond butter or ½ cup raw almonds

¼ cup tomato-based no-salt-added or low-sodium pasta sauce

1 tablespoon balsamic vinegar

Pinch of chili powder

1 avocado, peeled and sliced

1 tomato, chopped

2 cups shredded lettuce

2 cups shredded spinach

½ cup thinly sliced red onion

PER SERVING: CALORIES 270; PROTEIN 8g; CARBOHYDRATES 30g; TOTAL FAT 14.8g; SATURATED FAT 1.4g; CHOLESTEROL 0.3mg; SODIUM 138mg; FIBER 8.2g; BETA-CAROTENE 2,923mcg; VITAMIN C 12mg; CALCIUM 89mg; IRON 2.7mg; FOLATE 76mcg; MAGNESIUM 74mg; ZINC 1mg; SELENIUM 1.1mcg

Pita Stuffed with Seasoned Greens

SERVES 1

5–6 large leaves kale, Swiss chard, or mustard greens, tough stems removed

1 teaspoon lemon juice

Dash of garlic powder

1 (100% whole grain) pita

2 thin slices red onion

Sliced tomato

Low-sodium mustard (optional)

For a quick and portable lunch or dinner, stuff a whole grain pita with sautéed greens, red onion, and tomato.

Steam greens until tender, about 10–15 minutes. Sprinkle with lemon juice and garlic powder.

Stuff whole grain pita with greens, red onion, and tomato. Add mustard if desired.

You can also top this sandwich with your favorite healthful salad dressing.

PER SERVING: CALORIES 175; PROTEIN 8g; CARBOHYDRATES 35g; TOTAL FAT 2g; SATURATED FAT 0.2g; SODIUM 330mg; FIBER 7.1g; BETA-CAROTENE 9,654mcg; VITAMIN C 122mg; CALCIUM 141mg; IRON 3.2mg; FOLATE 49mcg; MAGNESIUM 52mg; ZINC 0.7mg; SELENIUM 6.1mcg

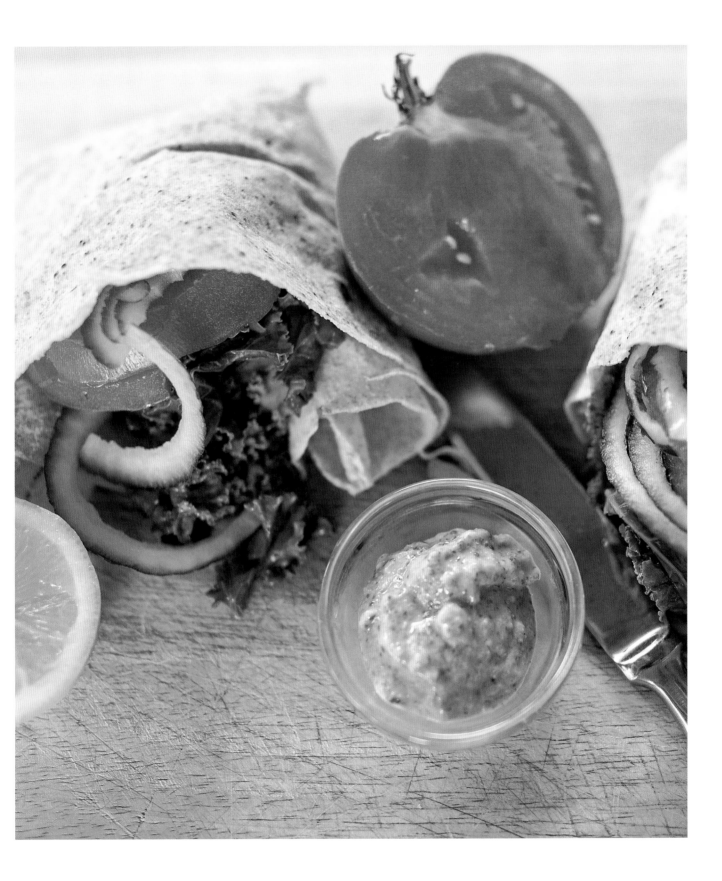

DESSERTS

There's no need to give up satisfying,
delicious desserts with the Nutritarian diet.

It is possible to create nutritious and tasty treats using only healthy, whole food ingredients. You can combine fresh, frozen, or unsulfured dried fruit; raw nuts and seeds; and whole grains to create simple but company-worthy treats.

Avoid refined sweets—including sugar, honey, corn syrup, agave nectar, maple syrup, and molasses—because they are low in nutrients and fiber and are rapidly absorbed by the body. More and more studies show that the consumption of these sweeteners, white sugar, and white flour products contributes significantly to the development of obesity, diabetes, heart disease, and certain cancers.

It is amazing that the conservative use of dried fruits, such as dates, can make desserts taste even better than conventional sweeteners, yet because of the nutrients and fibers they contain, those dried fruits prevent a dangerous sugar spike in the bloodstream.

Banana Oatmeal Cookies

SERVES 12

2 cups old-fashioned oats

1 teaspoon baking soda

1 teaspoon cinnamon

¼ teaspoon nutmeg

¼ teaspoon ground ginger

4 medium ripe bananas

¼ cup raw sunflower seeds

⅓ cup raisins or currants

These cookies add the perfect finish to brown bag lunches and are even great for a fast breakfast.

Preheat the oven to 300°F. Line a baking sheet with parchment or spray with nonstick spray.

Use a high-powered blender to process the oats into the consistency of flour. Pour the oat flour into a mixing bowl and add the baking soda, cinnamon, nutmeg, and ginger.

Blend the bananas in the blender until completely smooth. Add to the oat mixture along with the sunflower seeds and raisins or currants, and mix until well combined.

Use a 1-ounce cookie scoop (equal to about 2 tablespoons) to place spoonfuls of the cookie dough on the baking sheet. Dip the scoop in water to keep the dough from sticking. Use lightly moistened fingers to flatten each cookie slightly. Bake 15 minutes.

Cool cookies on a wire rack and store in an airtight container.

Makes about 24 cookies.

PER SERVING: CALORIES 115; PROTEIN 3g; CARBOHYDRATES 22g; TOTAL FAT 2.7g; SATURATED FAT 0.4g; SODIUM 106mg; FIBER 2.9g; BETA-CAROTENE 11mcg; VITAMIN C 4mg; CALCIUM 9mg; IRON 3.7mg; FOLATE 15mcg; MAGNESIUM 22mg; ZINC 0.2mg; SELENIUM 2mcg

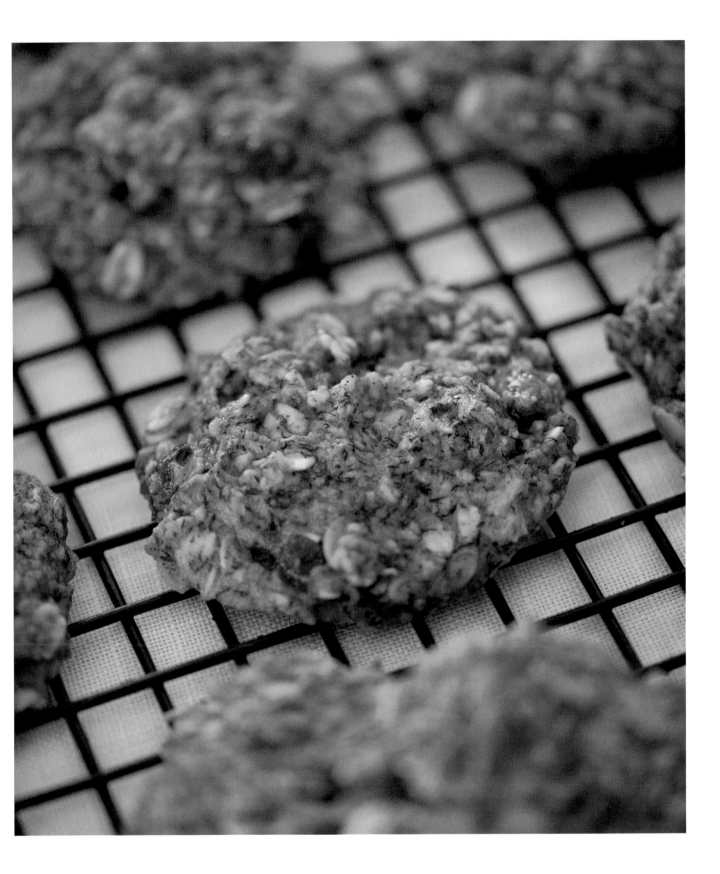

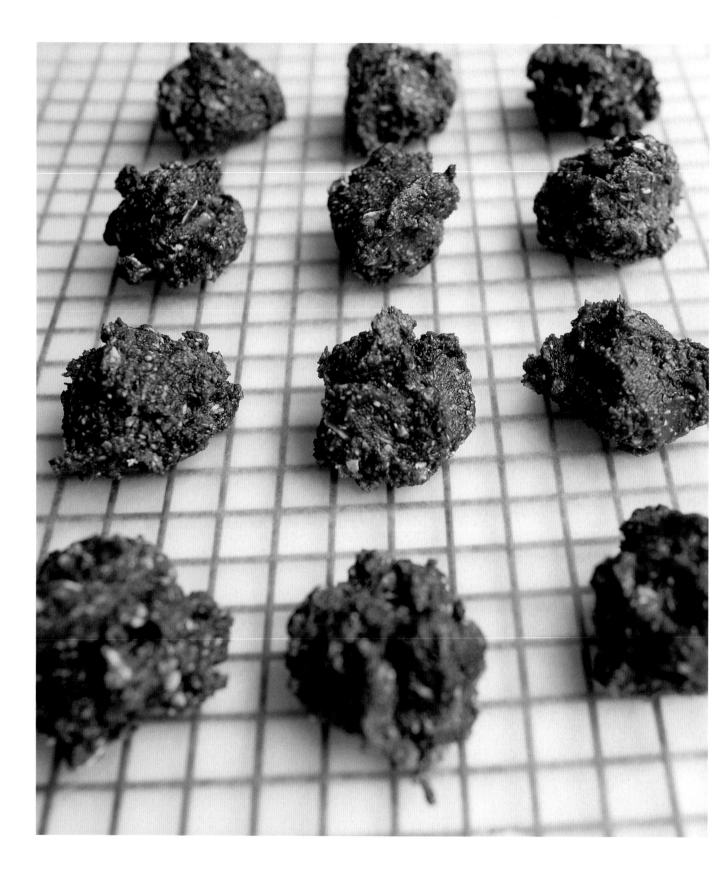

Chocolate Cherry Cookies

Preheat oven to 350°F.

Add dates to a food processor and pulse until they are blended and start to form a ball. Add the banana and almond butter and process until well combined.

Add oats, almond flour, cocoa powder, and vanilla extract and process until mixture forms a dough. If mixture is too wet, add more oats to adjust consistency. Add dried cherries and pulse again until just mixed. Chill dough for 10 minutes.

Drop by tablespoons onto a lightly oiled or parchment-lined cookie sheet. Bake 15–17 minutes.

Makes about 24 cookies.

SERVES 12

¾ cup dates, soaked for 15 minutes in warm water, then drained

1 very ripe banana

2 tablespoons raw almond or cashew butter

1 cup old-fashioned oats

½ cup almond flour (purchased or ground from raw almonds)

2 tablespoons natural cocoa powder

1 teaspoon alcohol-free vanilla or almond extract

½ cup chopped unsweetened dried cherries

PER SERVING: CALORIES 120; PROTEIN 3g; CARBOHYDRATES 21g; TOTAL FAT 3.9g; SATURATED FAT 0.6g; SODIUM 1mg; FIBER 2.7g; BETA-CAROTENE 3mcg; VITAMIN C 2mg; CALCIUM 20mg; IRON 0.8mg; FOLATE 10mcg; MAGNESIUM 47mg; ZINC 0.6mg; SELENIUM 3.2mcg

Chocolate Walnut Clusters

SERVES 14

2 large apples, peeled and sliced

2 teaspoons alcohol-free vanilla extract

1 cup pitted, chopped dates

⅔ cup whole wheat flour

1 ¼ teaspoons arrowroot powder

⅔ cup raw walnuts, ground

4 tablespoons natural cocoa powder

¾ cup old-fashioned oats

¾ cup chopped walnuts

....

Note: These cookies freeze well. For a chocolate coconut cookie, add 3 tablespoons unsweetened, shredded coconut.

Preheat oven to 375°F.

Blend apples, vanilla, and dates in a high-powered blender until creamy.

In a large bowl, combine the flour, arrowroot powder, ground nuts, and cocoa powder. Add the blended wet ingredients to the dry ingredients, and mix well. Stir in oats and chopped nuts.

Drop spoonfuls of cookie dough onto a lightly oiled or parchment-lined baking sheet. Bake 10 minutes.

Makes about 42 small cookies.

PER SERVING: CALORIES 151; PROTEIN 3g; CARBOHYDRATES 21g; TOTAL FAT 7.3g; SATURATED FAT 0.8g; SODIUM 1mg; FIBER 3.5g; BETA-CAROTENE 7mcg; VITAMIN C 1mg; CALCIUM 20mg; IRON 1.9mg; FOLATE 15mcg; MAGNESIUM 37mg; ZINC 0.6mg; SELENIUM 4.6mcg

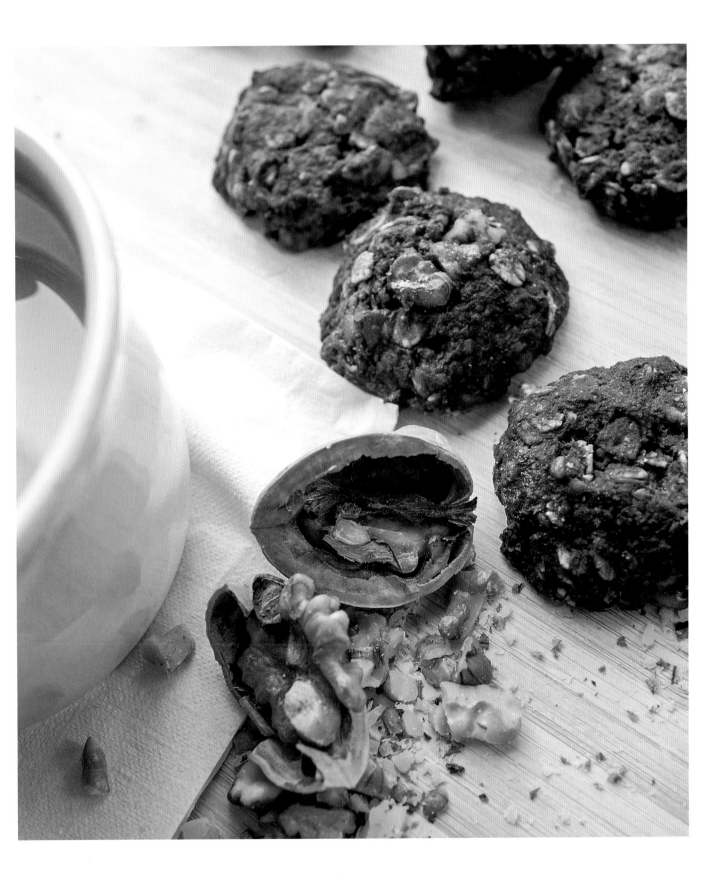

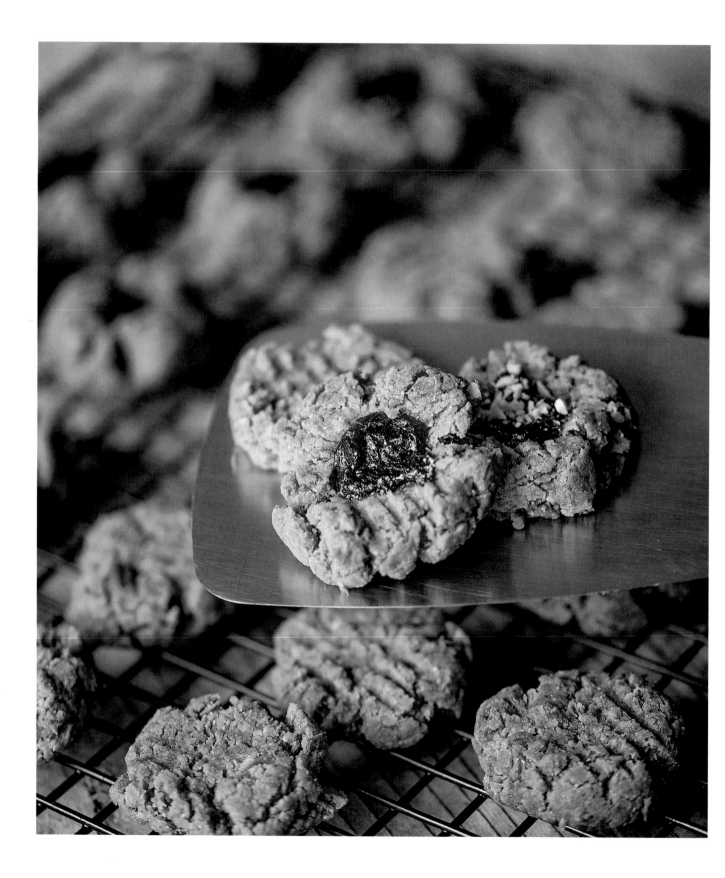

Peanut Butter Cookies

These Nutritarian cookies are made with cooked lentils instead of flour.

Preheat oven to 350°F.

Puree lentils in a high-powered blender. Place in a bowl and mix in ½ cup peanut butter.

Add the remaining ½ cup peanut butter to the blender, along with the dates and raisins, and blend until mixture is smooth and well combined. Remove from blender and combine with lentil/peanut butter mixture. Stir in baking powder and vanilla extract.

Roll into 1-inch balls and place on a nonstick baking mat or parchment-lined baking sheet. Bake 12 minutes, then press down with a fork. Bake an additional 20–25 minutes.

Cool completely on a wire rack. Store in refrigerator.

Makes 2 ½ dozen cookies.

SERVES 15

1 ½ cups cooked green lentils

1 cup natural, unsalted peanut butter, divided

6 medjool dates or 12 regular dates, pitted

½ cup raisins

1 tablespoon low-sodium baking powder

1 tablespoon alcohol-free vanilla extract

Note: If desired, before baking, make an indentation in the top of each cookie and add 1 teaspoon all-fruit preserves.

PER SERVING: CALORIES 164; PROTEIN 6g; CARBOHYDRATES 19g; TOTAL FAT 8.3g; SATURATED FAT 1.2g; SODIUM 3mg; FIBER 3.7g; BETA-CAROTENE 10mcg; CALCIUM 65mg; IRON 1.3mg; FOLATE 62mcg; MAGNESIUM 43mg; ZINC 0.9mg; SELENIUM 1.8mcg

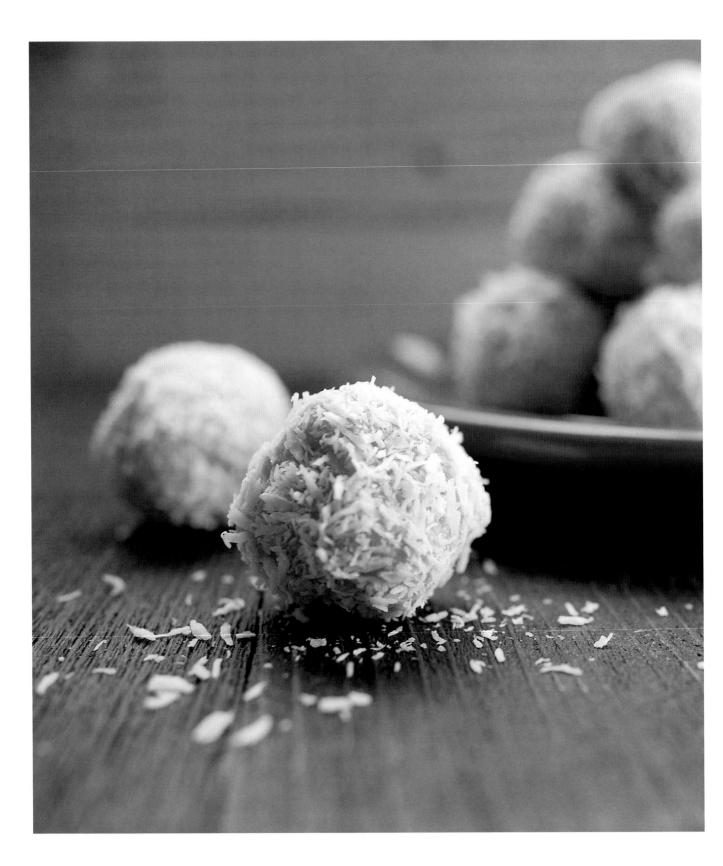

Lemon Balls

These bite-size treats are perfect for sharing with friends and family.

Place cashews in a food processor and process to a fine powder. Add lemon juice, lemon zest, coconut, and dates and process until consistency is thick and moist, adding a bit of water if needed.

Using hands, roll into small bite-size balls and then roll into some extra shredded coconut to coat the ball. Place into a container/dish and put in the refrigerator or freezer until hard.

Makes about 30 balls.

SERVES 15

2 cups raw cashews

2 organic lemons, juiced and zested

1 ½ cups unsweetened shredded coconut, plus extra for rolling

½ cup dates, pitted

PER SERVING: CALORIES 177; PROTEIN 4g; CARBOHYDRATES 12g; TOTAL FAT 13.9g; SATURATED FAT 6.6g; SODIUM 6mg; FIBER 2.7g; BETA-CAROTENE 1mcg; VITAMIN C 4mg; CALCIUM 13mg; IRON 1.6mg; FOLATE 7mcg; MAGNESIUM 64mg; ZINC 1.3mg; SELENIUM 5.5mcg

Chocolate Almond Truffles

SERVES 10

1 cup pitted dates

½ cup raw almond butter

2 tablespoons natural cocoa powder

3 tablespoons ground chia seeds

Natural cocoa powder, raw almonds or hazelnuts, or unsweetened shredded coconut

Add all ingredients to a food processor and blend until very well combined.

Remove from food processor and form into one-inch-diameter balls. Roll balls in cocoa powder, ground almonds or hazelnuts, or unsweetened shredded coconut.

Makes about 20 balls.

PER SERVING: CALORIES 136; PROTEIN 4g; CARBOHYDRATES 15g; TOTAL FAT 8.1g; SATURATED FAT 0.7g; SODIUM 2mg; FIBER 3.9g; BETA-CAROTENE 1mcg; CALCIUM 70mg; IRON 1mg; FOLATE 10mcg; MAGNESIUM 57mg; ZINC 0.7mg; SELENIUM 2.6mcg

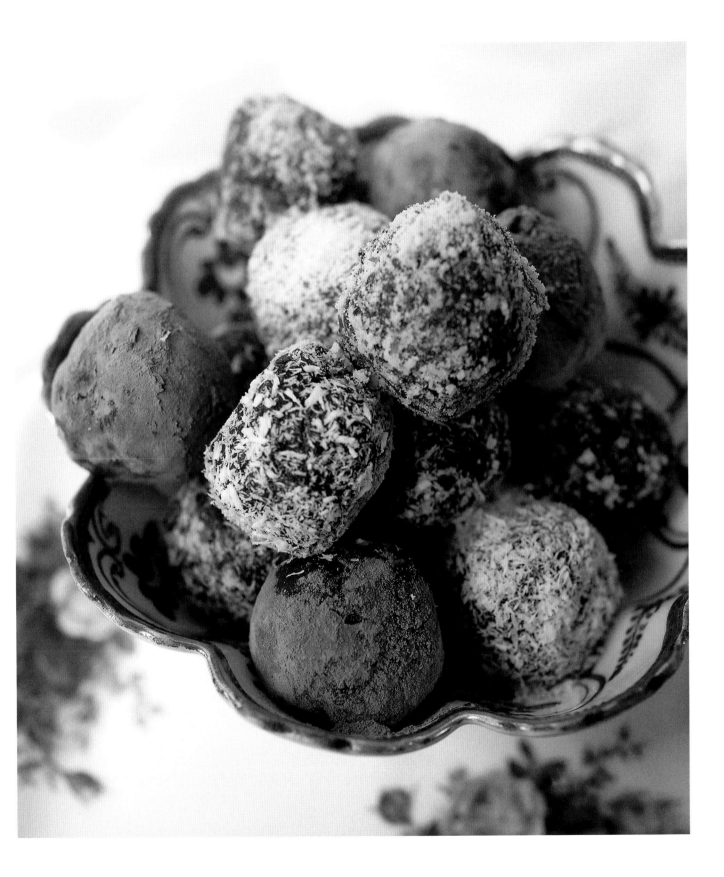

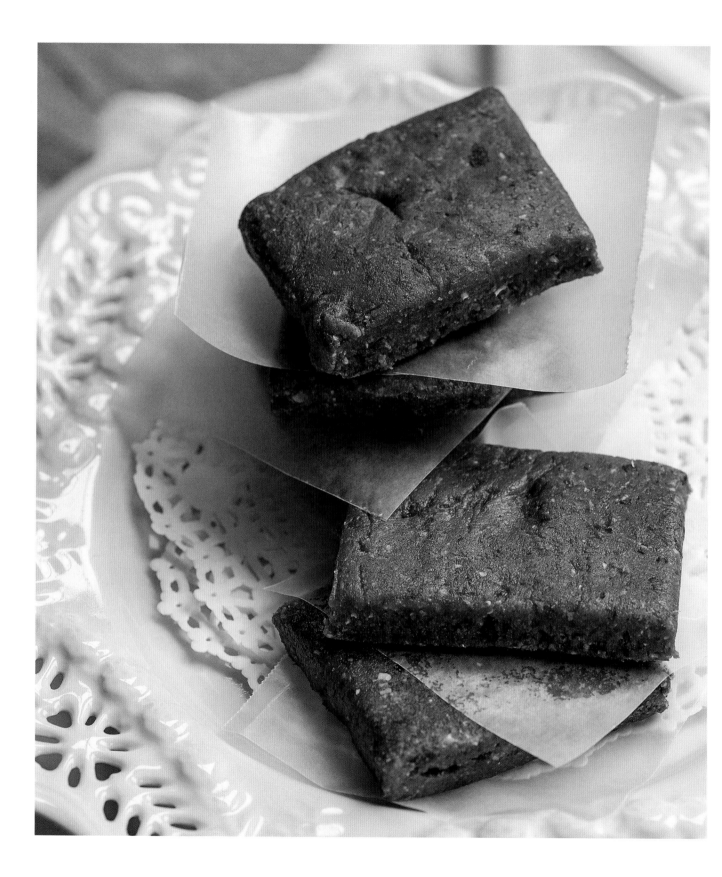

No-Bake Apricot Oat Bars

Soak apricots in nondairy milk for 1 hour.

In a food processor, process oats until coarsely chopped. Remove and set aside.

Place nuts, sunflower seeds, and flaxseed in food processor and chop into small pieces. Remove and add to chopped oats.

Add dates and cashew butter to food processor and process until very well combined and smooth. Mixture will start to form a ball. Add oat and nut mixture back to food processor along with soaked, drained apricot pieces and cinnamon, and combine.

Press mixture into an 8-by-8-inch baking pan. Make sure it is well compacted. Cut into bars.

SERVES 12

½ cup unsulfured dried apricots, chopped

⅓ cup unsweetened soy, hemp, or almond milk

¾ cup old-fashioned oats

1 cup raw cashews and/or almonds

2 tablespoons raw sunflower seeds

1 teaspoon ground flaxseed

1 cup dates, pitted

⅓ cup raw cashew butter

1 teaspoon cinnamon

PER SERVING: CALORIES 185; PROTEIN 5g; CARBOHYDRATES 22g; TOTAL FAT 10.4g; SATURATED FAT 1.6g; SODIUM 3mg; FIBER 3.2g; BETA-CAROTENE 119mcg; CALCIUM 35mg; IRON 1.5mg; FOLATE 20mcg; MAGNESIUM 75mg; ZINC 1.2mg; SELENIUM 4.7mcg

Chocolate "Cream" Pie

SERVES 8

For the crust

½ cup unsweetened shredded coconut

1 cup chopped raw macadamia nuts

16 pitted regular dates or 8 pitted medjool dates

For the filling

12 pitted regular dates or 6 pitted medjool dates*

2 avocados, peeled and pitted

½ cup raw cashews

4 tablespoons natural, nonalkalized cocoa powder

....

* Add more dates for a sweeter filling.

This pie is perfect for a special occasion. Avocados make the filling rich and creamy.

For the crust, combine the coconut, macadamia nuts, and dates in a food processor and process until well blended. Press the mixture into a glass pie pan.

For the filling, blend dates, avocado, cashews, and cocoa powder in a high-powered blender or food processor until creamy.

Spoon filling into crust and place in the freezer for 1 hour before serving.

> PER SERVING: CALORIES 422; PROTEIN 5g; CARBOHYDRATES 54g; TOTAL FAT 25g; SATURATED FAT 6.1g; SODIUM 7mg; FIBER 9.6g; BETA-CAROTENE 65mcg; VITAMIN C 3mg; CALCIUM 61mg; IRON 2.5mg; FOLATE 45mcg; MAGNESIUM 104mg; ZINC 1.4mg; SELENIUM 3.9mcg

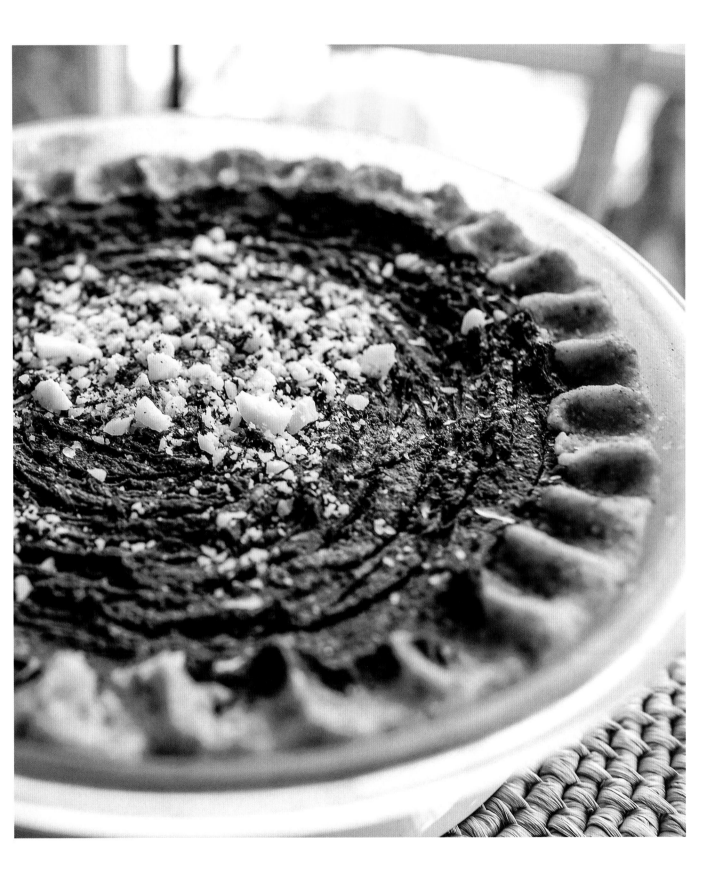

Berry Banana Compote

SERVES 2

1 banana

¼ cup unsweetened soy, hemp, or almond milk

1 cup frozen mixed berries

A few drops of alcohol-free vanilla extract

Dash of cinnamon

A delicious dessert before you know it: Combine five ingredients and microwave!

Mash banana with nondairy milk in a small microwave-safe bowl. Stir in berries and vanilla. Sprinkle with cinnamon. Microwave for about 1 minute.

Serve warm.

TIP: Berries and cherries are rich in flavonoids, compounds that are concentrated in their skins and are responsible for their red, blue, and purple colors. Flavonoids have antioxidant and anti-inflammatory benefits and help to support your nervous system and your overall health.

PER SERVING: CALORIES 81; PROTEIN 1g; CARBOHYDRATES 21g; TOTAL FAT 0.3g; SATURATED FAT 0.1g; SODIUM 2mg; FIBER 3.2g; BETA-CAROTENE 36mcg; VITAMIN C 36mg; CALCIUM 17mg; IRON 0.7mg; FOLATE 24mcg; MAGNESIUM 24mg; ZINC 0.2mg; SELENIUM 1.1mcg

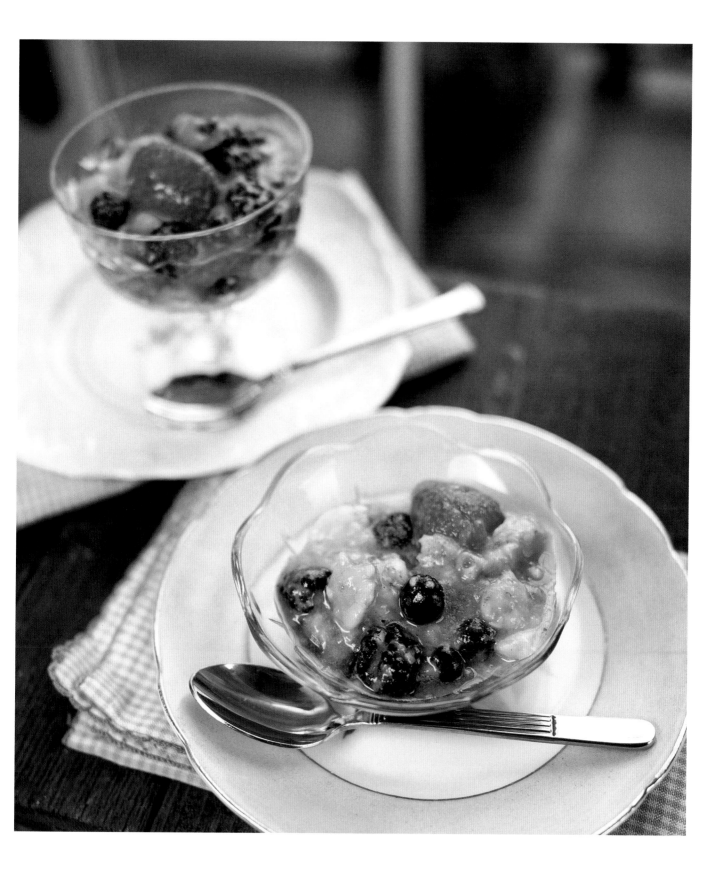

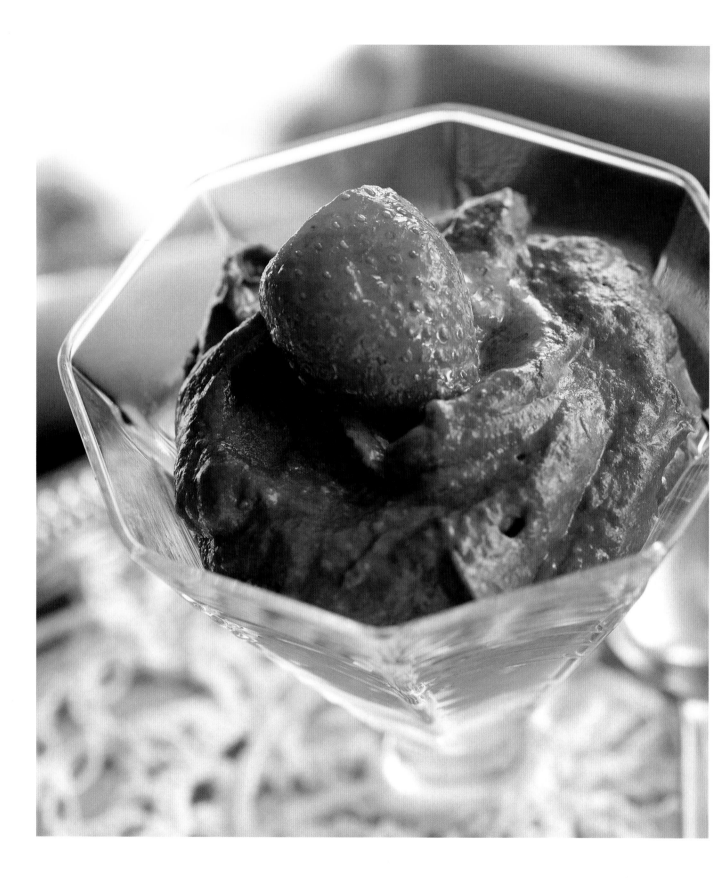

Chocolate Peanut Butter Pudding

Blend all ingredients in a food processor or high-powered blender until smooth and creamy. Add additional nondairy milk if needed to adjust consistency.

Divide into serving dishes and refrigerate for at least 2 hours.

SERVES 4

1 ripe banana

1 ripe avocado

½ cup natural, unsalted peanut butter

⅓ cup natural cocoa powder

4–6 regular dates or 2–3 medjool dates, pitted

¼ cup unsweetened soy, hemp, or almond milk

1 teaspoon alcohol-free vanilla extract

PER SERVING: CALORIES 322; PROTEIN 10g; CARBOHYDRATES 30g; TOTAL FAT 22g; SATURATED FAT 3.5g; SODIUM 12mg; FIBER 8.8g; BETA-CAROTENE 40mcg; VITAMIN C 6mg; CALCIUM 59mg; IRON 2.2mg; FOLATE 85mcg; MAGNESIUM 117mg; ZINC 1.9mg; SELENIUM 3.8mcg

Chocolate Chia Pudding

SERVES 4

2 cups unsweetened vanilla soy, hemp, or almond milk

4 medjool dates or 8 regular dates, pitted

3 tablespoons natural cocoa powder

½ teaspoon alcohol-free vanilla extract

½ cup chia seeds, divided

Blend milk, dates, cocoa powder, vanilla, and 2 tablespoons chia seeds in a high-powered blender. Stir in remaining chia seeds.

Refrigerate for 15 minutes and stir again to distribute seeds evenly.

If desired, top with fresh berries.

PER SERVING: CALORIES 200; PROTEIN 6g; CARBOHYDRATES 30g; TOTAL FAT 8.6g; SATURATED FAT 1g; SODIUM 98mg; FIBER 10.3g; BETA-CAROTENE 21mcg; CALCIUM 413mg; IRON 2.9mg; FOLATE 6mcg; MAGNESIUM 114mg; ZINC 1.4mg; SELENIUM 12.3mcg

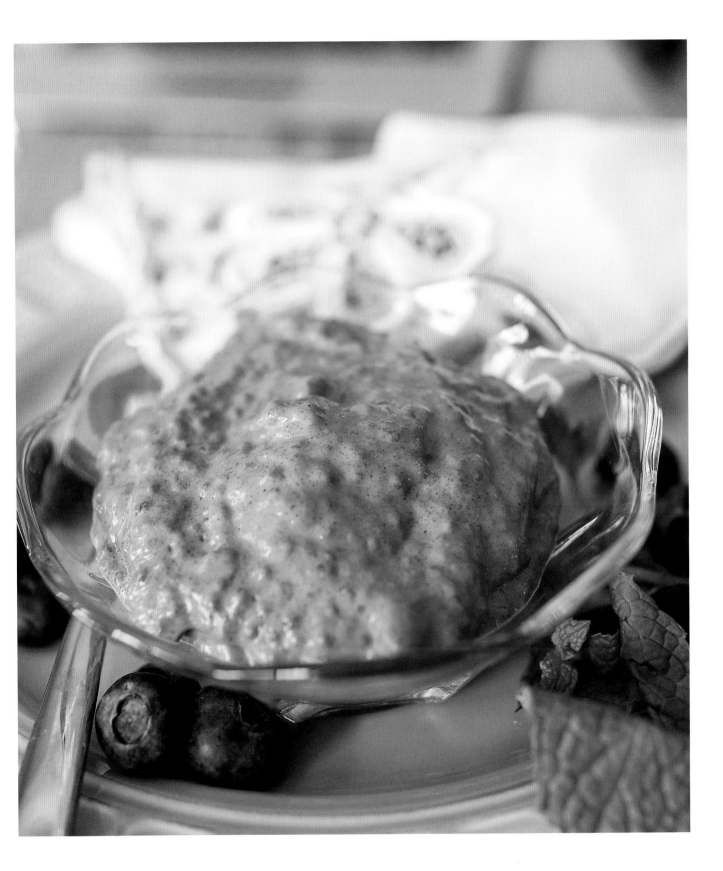

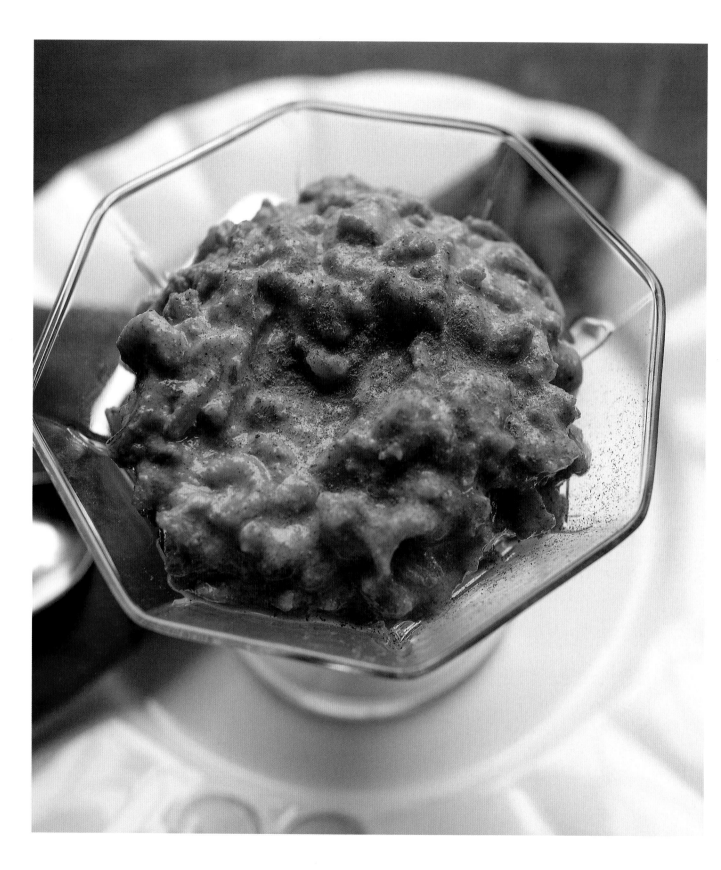

Easy Slow Cooker Rice Pudding

The aromas of cinnamon, vanilla, and cardamom will fill your home while this rice pudding is cooking.

Using a high-powered blender, blend dates with 4 cups nondairy milk.

Wipe the inside of a slow cooker with a small amount of olive oil. Place blended date mixture, the other 4 cups of milk, and remaining ingredients in the slow cooker and stir to combine.

Set the slow cooker on high until mixture starts to simmer, then reduce setting to low and cook 6–7 hours or until rice is tender. Discard cinnamon stick.

Remove from the slow cooker and place in a glass container. Chill in refrigerator until ready to serve. Pudding will thicken as it cools.

SERVES 6

6 medjool dates or 12 regular dates, pitted

8 cups soy, hemp, or almond milk, divided

1 cup uncooked wild rice

1 (2-inch) cinnamon stick

1 teaspoon alcohol-free vanilla extract

½ teaspoon ground cardamom

PER SERVING: CALORIES 344; PROTEIN 15g; CARBOHYDRATES 59g; TOTAL FAT 6.2g; SATURATED FAT 0.7g; SODIUM 169mg; FIBER 5.1g; BETA-CAROTENE 31mcg; CALCIUM 109mg; IRON 3.1mg; FOLATE 88mcg; MAGNESIUM 143mg; ZINC 2.1mg; SELENIUM 16.5mcg

Pumpkin Pie Mousse

SERVES 3

1 cup pumpkin puree*

½ cup soy, hemp, or almond milk (adjust to desired consistency)

3 medjool dates or 6 regular dates, pitted

½ cup cooked cannellini beans

½ teaspoon pumpkin pie spice

¼ teaspoon cinnamon

Toasted pecans, for garnish

....

Use fresh pumpkin puree or pumpkin puree packed in non-BPA cartons.

Blend all ingredients except pecans in a high-powered blender till well blended, light, and fluffy. Top with toasted pecans or if desired, a dollop of cashew cream.

To make cashew cream: Blend 1⅓ cups raw cashews; ¾ cup vanilla soy, hemp, or almond milk; and ⅔ cup pitted dates in a high-powered blender until smooth and creamy.

PER SERVING: CALORIES 142; PROTEIN 5g; CARBOHYDRATES 31g; TOTAL FAT 1g; SATURATED FAT 0.2g; SODIUM 22mg; FIBER 5.3g; BETA-CAROTENE 1,221mcg; VITAMIN C 4mg; CALCIUM 60mg; IRON 1.7mg; FOLATE 58mcg; MAGNESIUM 49mg; ZINC 0.6mg; SELENIUM 2.5mcg

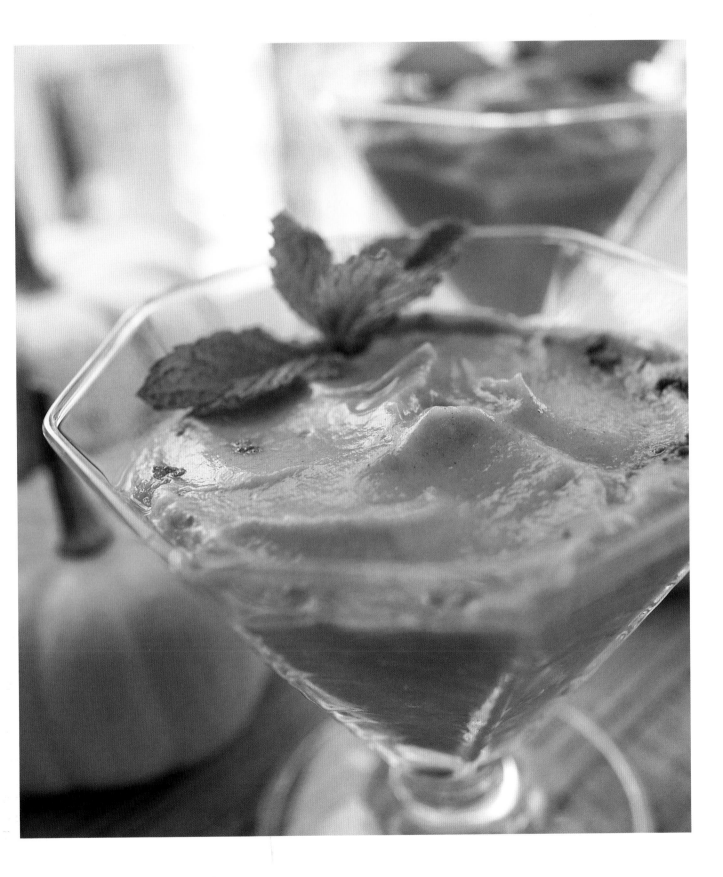

Vanilla Sabayon with Fresh Fruit

SERVES 8

1 ¾ cups raw cashews, soaked overnight

7 medjool dates or 14 regular dates, pitted

¼ to ½ cup coconut water, as needed

1 vanilla bean, pulp scraped out

½ teaspoon alcohol-free vanilla extract

Your choice of fruit

Sabayon is a custard-like dessert popular in southern France; it's also known as zabaglione in Italy. For this Nutritarian version, cashews, dates, and coconut water are blended with a fresh vanilla bean.

In a high-powered blender, combine all ingredients except for the fruit and blend until very smooth, adding more coconut water as needed to achieve a thick but pourable mixture.

For a nice presentation, alternate layers of fruit and sabayon in a clear parfait glass or just spoon over your choice of fresh fruit in a bowl.

PER SERVING: CALORIES 203; PROTEIN 5g; CARBOHYDRATES 24g; TOTAL FAT 11.3g; SATURATED FAT 2g; SODIUM 11mg; FIBER 2.3g; BETA-CAROTENE 19mcg; CALCIUM 25mg; IRON 1.9mg; FOLATE 10mcg; MAGNESIUM 88mg; ZINC 1.6mg; SELENIUM 5.2mcg

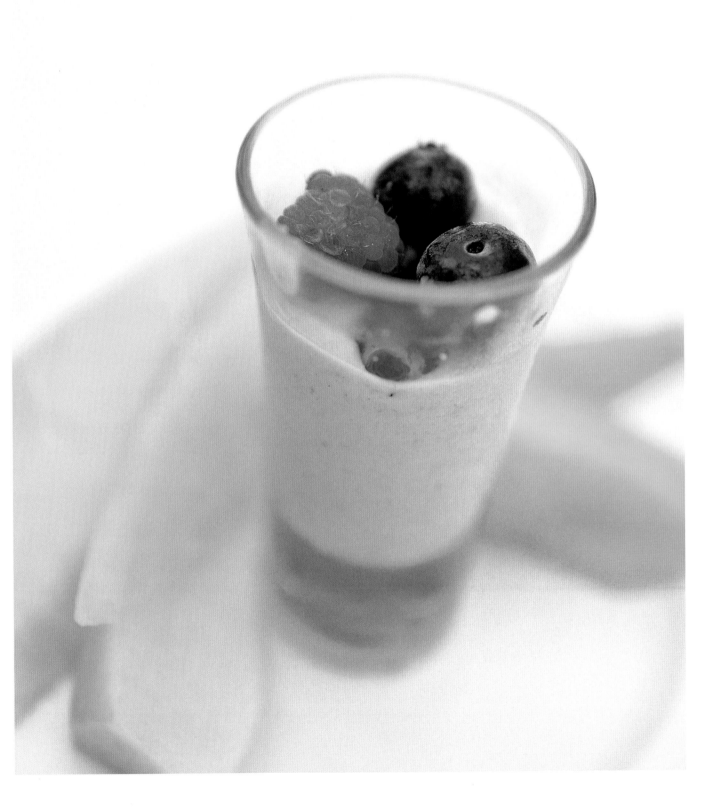

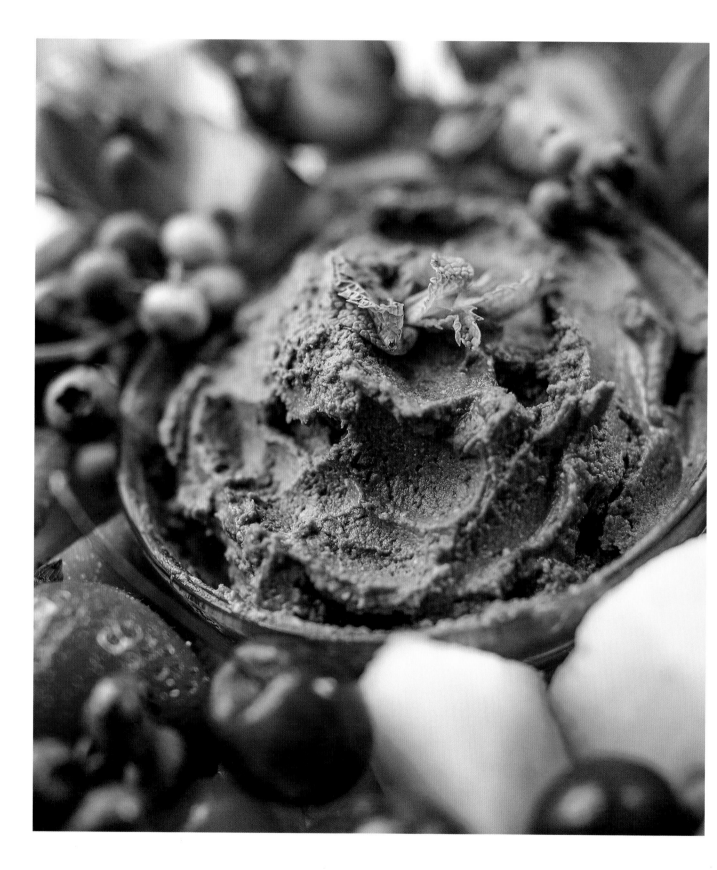

Chocolate Hummus

Serve with your favorite fresh fruit.

Place all ingredients in a high-powered blender or food processor and blend until very smooth. Add more nondairy milk if mixture is too thick. Chill thoroughly.

Hummus will thicken as it chills; you may need to thin it with a little more nondairy milk before serving with fresh fruit.

1 ½ cups cooked or 1 (15-ounce) can low-sodium or no-salt-added black beans, drained

4 medjool dates, pitted

¼ cup raw almonds

¼ cup natural cocoa powder

1 teaspoon alcohol-free vanilla extract

¼ teaspoon cinnamon

¼ cup soy, hemp, or almond milk

TIP: Delicious fruit sorbets or ice "creams" are quick and easy to make when using a good blender. They are a great way to healthfully satisfy your sweet tooth—and you can get creative with your favorite fruit combinations.

PER SERVING: CALORIES 151; PROTEIN 6g; CARBOHYDRATES 26g; TOTAL FAT 3.9g; SATURATED FAT 0.6g; SODIUM 7mg; FIBER 6.8g; BETA-CAROTENE 15mcg; CALCIUM 46mg; IRON 1.8mg; FOLATE 72mcg; MAGNESIUM 75mg; ZINC 1mg; SELENIUM 1.7mcg

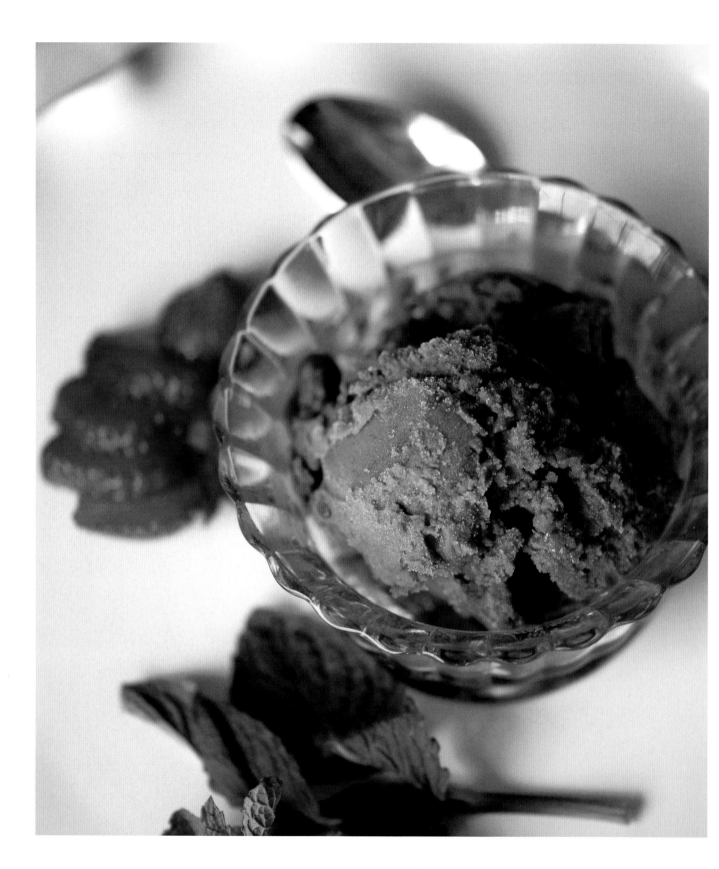

Five-Minute Chocolate Ice Cream

Add nondairy milk, vanilla, dates, and cocoa powder to a high-powered blender and start to blend. Drop frozen banana pieces in slowly. Add additional nondairy milk if needed to reach desired consistency.

If you like, blend in ¼ cup raw nuts—hazelnuts, macadamia nuts, cashews, almonds, or pecans—with the other ingredients.

SERVES 2

2 tablespoons soy, hemp, or almond milk

1 teaspoon vanilla

2 regular dates or 1 medjool date

1–2 tablespoons unsweetened cocoa powder

2 large bananas, frozen

TIP: Keep frozen bananas on hand so you are ready to whip up a good-for-you frozen dessert whenever the mood strikes. To freeze bananas, peel, cut in thirds, and seal in a plastic bag before freezing.

PER SERVING: CALORIES 175; PROTEIN 3g; CARBOHYDRATES 43g; TOTAL FAT 1.1g; SATURATED FAT 0.4g; SODIUM 10mg; FIBER 5.3g; BETA-CAROTENE 46mcg; VITAMIN C 12mg; CALCIUM 22mg; IRON 0.9mg; FOLATE 33mcg; MAGNESIUM 61mg; ZINC 0.5mg; SELENIUM 2.5mcg

Mango Macadamia Nut Ice Cream

SERVES 2

½ cup almond, hemp, or
soy milk (or more to achieve
desired consistency)

1 ripe banana, frozen

2 cups frozen mango

¼ cup raw macadamia nuts
or walnuts

Blend ingredients in a high-powered blender. Freeze until firm.

PER SERVING: CALORIES 305; PROTEIN 5g; CARBOHYDRATES 44g;
TOTAL FAT 14.6g; SATURATED FAT 2.4g; SODIUM 34mg; FIBER 6g;
BETA-CAROTENE 1,073mcg; VITAMIN C 65mg; CALCIUM 51mg;
IRON 1.4mg; FOLATE 96mcg; MAGNESIUM 69mg; ZINC 0.5mg;
SELENIUM 5.1mcg

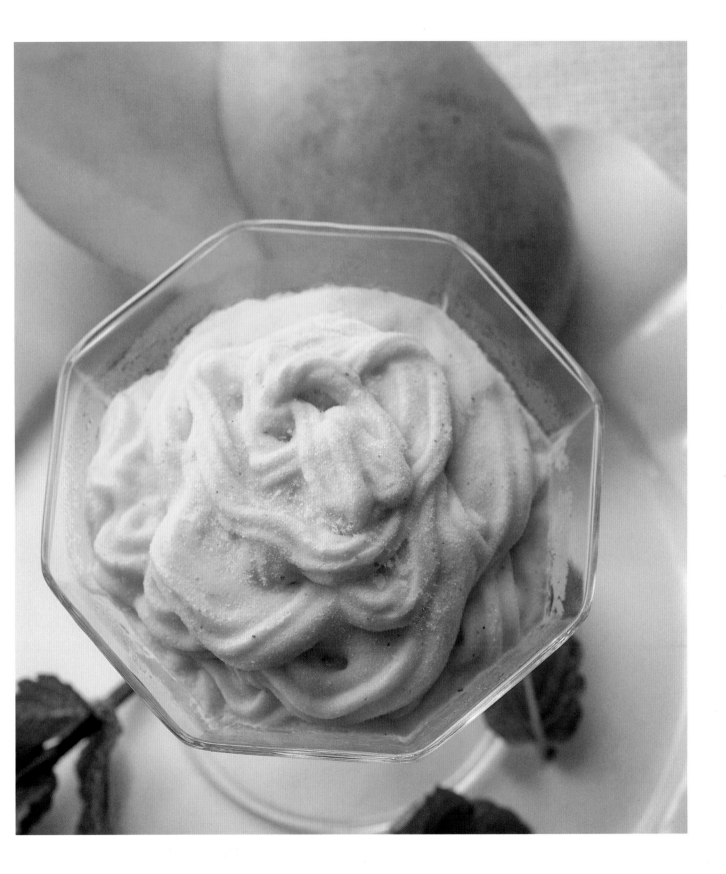

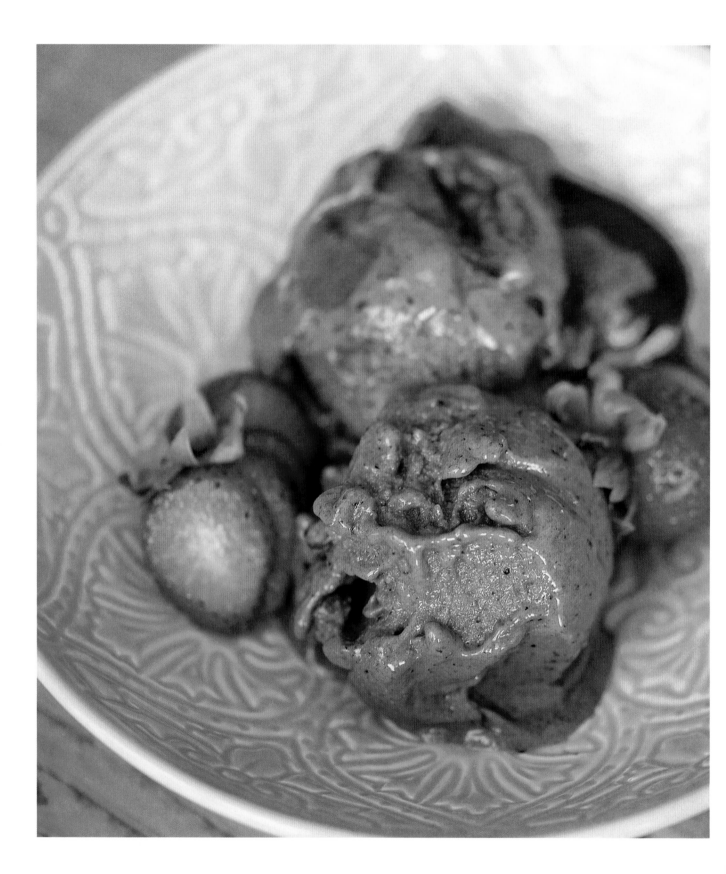

Mixed-Berry Freeze

This guilt-free dessert is a great way to get your daily serving of antioxidant-rich berries.

Blend ingredients in a high-powered blender until creamy.

SERVES 2

¼ cup soy, hemp, or almond milk

1 ripe banana, frozen

1 (10-ounce) package frozen mixed berries

2 tablespoons ground flaxseeds

PER SERVING: CALORIES 167; PROTEIN 4g; CARBOHYDRATES 33g; TOTAL FAT 4.2g; SATURATED FAT 0.4g; SODIUM 20mg; FIBER 7g; BETA-CAROTENE 55mcg; VITAMIN C 36mg; CALCIUM 45mg; IRON 1.4mg; FOLATE 40mcg; MAGNESIUM 62mg; ZINC 0.6mg; SELENIUM 4.4mcg

Acknowledgments

I want to thank and recognize my excellent supportive team at DrFuhrman.com that made this book possible. They include marketing director Heidi Pellegrini, who played an important role in organizing this project; Eileen Murphy for editing; art director Lauren Russell, and her team Tim Shay and Kyle Fidel. Meredith Russell also contributed to the photos and art. Linda Popescu, RD, and Mary Becker contributed to the recipes and Mary Becker also was the food stylist preparing and plating most of the recipes for the photography. The majority of the photos were taken by Kyle Fidel, Lisa Fuhrman, and Jenna Fuhrman.

International Conversion Chart

Oven temperature equivalents

Measurement equivalents
Measurements should always be level unless directed otherwise

Oven temperature equivalents	Measurement equivalents
250°F = 120°C	⅛ teaspoon = 0.5 ml
275°F = 135°C	¼ teaspoon = 1 ml
300°F = 150°C	½ teaspoon = 2 ml
325°F = 160°C	1 teaspoon = 5 ml
350°F = 180°C	1 tablespoon = 3 teaspoons = ½ fluid ounce = 15 ml
375°F = 190°C	2 tablespoons = ⅛ cup = 1 fluid ounce = 30 ml
400°F = 200°C	4 tablespoons = ¼ cup = 2 fluid ounces = 60 ml
425°F = 220°C	5⅓ tablespoons = ⅓ cup = 3 fluid ounces = 80 ml
450°F = 230°C	8 tablespoons = ½ cup = 4 fluid ounces = 120 ml
475°F = 240°C	10⅔ tablespoons = ⅔ cup = 5 fluid ounces = 160 ml
500°F = 260°C	12 tablespoons = ¾ cup = 6 fluid ounces = 180 ml
	16 tablespoons = 1 cup = 8 fluid ounces = 240 ml

Index

Recipes are organized under recipe main ingredients. Consult the Table of Contents for an alphabetical list of the recipes. Page references followed by *p* indicate a photograph.

LDL (low-density lipoprotein) cholesterol, 7

leeks, 38p

legumes: lentils and split peas as, 6; resistant starch and fiber of, 6

lemon juice, 14. *See also specific recipes*

lemons: Chopped Nutty Fruit and Vegetable Salad, 99p; Lemon Balls, 254p–55; Lemony Mushroom Quinoa, 208p–9

lentils: Carrot and Red Lentil Soup, 120p–21; Gingery Red Lentil Butternut Soup, 126–27p; Peach and Leafy Lentil Salad, 88–89p; Peanut Butter Cookies, 252p–53; resistant starch of, 6

lettuce: Peach and Leafy Lentil Salad red leaf, 88–89p; Tomato Almond Pocket Pitas, 240p–41. *See also* romaine lettuce

lime juice, 14. *See also specific recipes*

lycopene carotenoid, 8, 157

macadamia nuts, 278–79p

main dish recipes: burgers, pizzas, and wraps, 218p–23, 226–43p; general, 151–202p; non-vegan, 212–25p; quick whole grain, 203–11p; a word about, 150, 203, 212

mangos: Kale and Fruit Salad with Almond Citrus Dressing, 96–97p; Mango Macadamia Nut Ice Cream, 278–79p; Peach and Leafy Lentil Salad, 88–89p

MatoZest, 14, 113p, 118–19p

mayonnaise: Better-for-You "Mayo," 70p–71; how to make homemade healthy, 238

meat dishes: Chicken-Seasoned Quinoa, 214–15p; fats in animal products of, 4, 7; Stuffed Peppers with Mushrooms, Greens, and Ground Turkey, 224–25p. *See also* burgers

micronutrients, 5–6

milk (whole), 7

mushrooms: Black Bean, Beef, and Mushroom Burgers, 218p–19; Chicken-Seasoned Quinoa, 214–15p; Creamy Polenta with Mushrooms, Kale, and Chickpeas, 162–63p; Easy Split Pea Stew, 124p–25; Easy Vegetable Pizza, 222p–23; as G-BOMBS superfood, 9; health benefits of, 8, 125; Japanese Curry Stir Fry, 194–95p; Lemony Mushroom Quinoa, 208p–9; Mushroom and Barley Soup, 128p–29; Mushroom Kale Bean Pasta, 182–83p; Mushroom, Onion, and Pesto Pizza, 232p–33; Old-Fashioned Grain and Mushroom Salad, 82–83p; Quick Fish and White Bean Stew, 216p–17; Ready-in-a-Flash Mushroom Soup, 140p–41; Stuffed Peppers with Mushrooms, Greens, and Ground Turkey, 224–25p; Sweet Potato Stuffed Mushrooms, 188p–89

mustard greens: health benefits of, 5; Pita Stuffed with Seasoned Greens, 242–43p

myrosinase enzyme, 5

nut allergies, 8

nut-based dressings. *See* salad dressings

nutrients: fruit, 6–7; health benefits of plant-derived, 2; micronutrients, 5; phytonutrients, 2; vegetables, 5–6, 8, 10, 14

Nutritarian diet: basic guidelines of the lifestyle, 4; description and health benefits of a, 1–2; foods that make up the foundations of, 5–10; the results that you'll experience with a, 3

Nutri-tella, 110–11p

nuts: health benefits of, 7–8, 33; as olive oil alternative, 7. *See also specific type of nut*

oatmeal: Banana Oatmeal Cookies, 246–47p; Blue Apple Nut Oatmeal, 18p–19; Chia Seed Breakfast Pudding, 30–31p; Cinnamon-Spiced Baked, 22–23p; Hot Oatmeal Smoothie, 41p; No-Bake Apricot Oat Bars, 258p–59; No-Cook Strawberry Oatmeal To-Go, 20p–21; steel cut oats (Scotch or Irish oats), 18p–21

olive oil alternatives, 7

omega-3 fats, 8, 33

onions: health benefits of, 8, 125; one of the G-BOMBS superfoods, 9. *See also specific recipes*

orange juice: Balsamic Tomato and Asparagus Salad, 74p–75; Orange Pomegranate Sparkler, 52–53p; Peach and Leafy Lentil Salad, 88–89p; Sweet Shredded Carrot Salad, 80p–81

oranges: Chopped Nutty Fruit and Vegetable Salad, 99p; Green Lemonade, 44p–45; Kale and Fruit Salad with Almond Citrus Dressing, 96–97p; Margarita Cooler, 50–51p; Orange Sesame Dressing, 62p; Super-Easy Blended Salad, 46p

parsley health benefits, 13

Peach and Leafy Lentil Salad, 88–89p

peanut butter: Chickpea Burgers, 228p–29; Chocolate Peanut Butter Pudding, 264p–65; Chocolate Peanut Butter Smoothie, 47p; Orange Sesame Dressing, 62p; Peanut Butter Cookies, 252p–53

peas: black-eyed, 6; Chicken-Seasoned Quinoa, 214–15p; Creamy Barley Risotto with Tomatoes and Peas, 204–5p; Easy Split Pea Stew, 124p–25; steaming snow, 11

pecans: Creamy Lemon Dressing, 61p; Pumpkin Pie Mousse, 270–71p

peppers: jalapeño, 76–77p; yellow and orange, 36p–37, 206p–7. *See also* green bell peppers; red bell peppers

phytochemicals, 5, 6, 21

phytonutrients, 2

pineapples: Hawaiian Tofu Stir Fry, 196p–97; Kale and Fruit Salad with Almond Citrus Dressing, 96–97p